Here's to you living out your AgePoten

Lo

D1035501

This book was **donated** to us.
Please treat it as the **gift** it is.
"Literature is my utopia."
~ Helen Keller

"Awak... ...est
of you... ...age. Lori Camp... ...e
profiles of happy, successful... ...u
choose to d... ...l

"The
emb
tenti

"[The co...
way. We
has an u
He accep
men. Not
tributors i...
gone about
forces, incl...

"Believe it or n...
filling life you
and her thriver

Awaken Your AgePotential

Awaken Your AgePotential

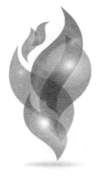

Exploring Chosen Paths of Thrivers

Lori Campbell

ISBN: 978-1-59298-508-1
Library of Congress Control Number: 2012948665

Printed in the United States of America
First Printing: 2013
17   16   15   14   13   5   4   3   2   1

Book design by Mayfly Design
Typeset in Adobe Caslon Pro

Beaver's Pond Press, Inc.
7108 Ohms Lane, Edina, MN 55439-2129
(952) 829-8818 • www.BeaversPondPress.com

To order, visit www.BeaversPondBooks.com
or call (800) 901-3480. Reseller discounts available.

This book is dedicated to all aspiring thrivers.

May you always remember you have inherent value and purpose regardless of your age. Embrace the new vision of aging set before you and have the courage, life meaning and joy to live out your...AgePotential™.

Contents

Acknowledgments

First and foremost, I thank God who made all things possible.

Among the many people who supported, inspired, and encouraged me in bringing this book to fruition, I must first acknowledge and thank each one of my contributing authors whose stories present the reader with profound depth of personal insight. I am forever grateful for their willingness to share their inner-most thoughts and experiences of thriving.

Thank you to the following individuals who without their contributions and support this book would not have been written: my publisher, Beaver's Pond Press; my editing team who was a great source of strength: Amy, Jessica, Angela, and Molly; Ryan, my graphic designer, for bringing AgePotential alive through his expressive design.

A heartfelt thank you to Jeremy Bloom for writing the foreword and all those who provided reviews and testimonials for my book.

To my mastermind group who helped keep my vision fresh and full of promise.

Most especially to my family and friends who so diligently walked along side of me and faithfully kept my enthusiasm stoked. Thank you!

Special thanks to all thrivers who are boldly living out their AgePotential and paving the way for the rest of us to follow suit. Your chosen way of life has forever changed the way I think and live and has affirmed my life work. It's a beautiful thing when a career and a passion come together. I celebrate my work as a labor of love. I am grateful to serve in this capacity.

Foreword

Human life is more than the process of aging. It is more than the process of living and dying, of working and retiring, of getting married and becoming widowed, of becoming a parent and sending adult children into the world. While the external experience is the content of life, the quality of the content is determined internally. Human life is about the experience within and how we respond to the external experiences.

If we choose to allow our identity to be statically defined by the external things in our lives (such as education, spouses, children, and careers), and those external things change, where is our identity? AgePotential—which means to live out our full potential at every age—depends on our *choice* to define ourselves by our internal attitude toward the ever-evolving experience of life, not by the external circumstances themselves.

Lori Campbell's *Awaken to Your AgePotential* is about the experience within each of us to live an evolving life true to our potential, regardless of what society tells us about our chronology. AgePotential is a movement redefining the way our culture views the concept of "age"—rather than defining our worth based on the number we're given on our birthday each year, AgePotential says we should view our worth on an individual level, each person choosing to identify it for themselves, and choosing to do so on an evolving basis.

The stories in this book share the secrets and values to living a life according to AgePotential. It wisely expounds these values through true stories of love, grief, humor, loss, philanthropy, work, and looking at it all through the lens of embracing change and choosing a life of fulfillment and satisfaction, taking that responsibility on as an internal journey rather than relying on external circumstances to bring us there.

This philosophy takes all focus off of our chronology while embracing it at the same time. It demands that we "live in the now," accepting and moving confidently into new stages and experiences of life with a spirit of resourcefulness, while always looking back at where we came from with a smile rather than a longing. It is a daily devotion and commitment to live this way, yet this attitude will be all the life *fulfillment* insurance that we'll ever need.

On a large scale, the concept of AgePotential can change our culture's attitude toward medicine, law, education, entertainment, media, etc. On a personal level, it changes how we approach every aspect of our lives—family, career, love, etc. The "thrivers" in this book give us the roadmap on how to respect the past, embrace the present, and look forward to the future— our responsibility for our future resting in our present. This book is much more than an awakening. It is the first spark of a revolution.

—Jeremy Bloom

Jeremy Bloom, former NFL Football player and two-time Olympic skier, is the founder of the nonprofit Jeremy Bloom's Wish of a Lifetime. This 501(c)3 foundation is a living memorial to his grandmother and grants wishes to individuals in their autumn years of life. He is also a cofounder of Integrate, a next-generation advertising marketplace that streamlines the media transaction process. Jeremy was named by Forbes as one of the "30 under 30" tech executives under the age of thirty making waves in the technology space.

Generation AgePotential:
The Next Generation

At one time, I used to think *thriving* older adults were either a select group of people with a rare set of genes or a group who had lived a life of entitlement. But the contrary is true. As a gerontologist and qualitative researcher, I've worked with countless older thrivers who adamantly claim to be just like you and me. While those who thrive might make the process of growing older look like a joyful adventure, through their stories I've learned they have all experienced and endured significant pain, loss, and hardship—just like the rest of us. What does set them apart, however, is the way they choose to perceive and respond to the world.

They not only personify the latest research on aging and a concept called epigenetics, which I will discuss later on in the book, but they also embody what I'm calling AgePotential, a new way to think about the aging process that will help everyone—no matter their chronological age or genetic makeup—live a more fulfilling, rich, and giving life.

Before I introduce the idea of AgePotential, let's take a closer look at what sets thrivers and non-thrivers apart. Non-thrivers tend to embody the old paradigm of aging, which views the process of growing old as something that's fixed and mechanical, or in other words, as something that "just happens to you." Non-thrivers unwittingly believe—or choose to believe—they are victims of their genes, and they often take a passive approach to their aging journey. Sadly, it is common for them to die with untapped talent and unlived potential.

Thrivers, on the other hand, tend to embody the new paradigm of aging, in which "awareness" is a foundation to knowing the aging process is pliable. Thrivers believe they can influence how they age, so they take responsibility for their health and aging journey. These individuals do not follow the status quo; instead, they age with intention, live by design, and act on their passions and dreams. Thrivers expect to lead healthy and vibrant lives until they die.

The thriving adults I've had the opportunity to work with have made me aware of the difference between the two paradigms in ways research itself could not—and they have forever changed how I aspire to live and age. But the most startling realization I've made is that our ability to live healthy, passionate, and purposeful lives is not dictated by *age*, but rather by awareness, intention, and action. I believe many of these older adults are more aware of their potential to lead full, healthy, and significant lives than many of my peers and individuals in younger generations.

But why do non-thrivers lack that same awareness? Is it possible that Western society's obsession with youth has overshadowed the real potential of later life? I think so. Our preoccupation with youth is not only extremely detrimental to psyches of all ages, but it also denies a significant part of the human lifespan. By considering people in later life as one generalized group, the youth obsession has a tendency to make older individuals feel invisible. Denial causes ageist thinking, and we're left with a huge discrepancy between society's perception of growing old and the real possibility of aging to our potential. From my observations, the discrepancy remains strong despite the hard science and growing number of thriving older adults. Society's perception simply doesn't reflect the true possibility inherent in later life.

What's more, our society focuses relentlessly on disease and disability over wellness and prevention.

Why do we take on the victim mentality? When will we tire of waiting for malady and instead shift our focus to prevention? Research shows that one of the most pervasive barriers to shifting our collective focus from disease management to prevention is the perpetuation of the deception that aging is a continual downward spiral, both mentally and physically. People continue to associate disease to age. Aging is not a disease. Aging is not a disability. People of all ages encounter disease and disability.

True, our chronological age is nonnegotiable, but our psychological age—how we think and feel about ourselves—is something we *can* change. And our ability to recognize this fact holds the most promise for erasing the discrepancy and discovering the true potential yet to be unleashed within us all. As a gerontologist, I have found older adults to be a viable source of firsthand knowledge on the fundamental factors of well-being, and I view them as experts on their lives and the aging process. As such, these older thrivers deserve more attention. Their life stories will awaken the world and show the possibility of maintaining and enhancing overall health throughout the course of a lifetime. The current lack of awareness of the "thriving possibility" is not due to a lack of role models but to the role models' general lack of visibility. In my field, the norm is to study older adults, collect data, and share the results in a highly impersonal way. But I believe the possibility of AgePotential cannot be fully or accurately portrayed through a statistic. We need to hear thrivers' stories from a first-person point of view—that's where the awakening will come from.

Thrivers present the possibility of aging with a sense of purpose, a zest for life, a strong constitution, and independence. And by leading through example, they also extend an invitation for us to do the same, no matter our DNA makeup or genetic code. The insight I gained through my relationships with people who live their lives (in the words of my eighty-six-year-old friend) at "full tilt" led to my "aha" moment—the moment I discovered that my calling as a gerontologist is to bring their empowering message about aging to the world. It was never my life ambition to become an entrepreneur, but passion drives you to places you never expect to go. So, inspired by these thriving older adults, I launched Gen AP, LLC, to develop a new concept of aging and transform how the world grows older. My belief is that we all have the power to thrive in our own unique way—we just need to awaken to the potential first.

My personal awakening has been an ongoing journey, but meeting one person in particular seemed to pique my curiosity about these thriving older adults: I met Verra while administrating a qualitative research study on centenarians. She lived in a retirement community with other "independent dwellers." Verra, then 101 years old, had a vivacious personality and an expressive sense of style. "I love to get all dolled up," she told me. One of her style trademarks was to wear a bow in her hair that matched her outfit. According to Verra, going to the community dining room for dinner was like attending a party, so she had to be sure she wore just the right amount of rouge and lipstick. Once at the dining room, greeting everyone who came for dinner was something Verra took seriously. She felt useful and needed, and she was.

During childhood, Sunday dinners and singing played a significant role in Verra's life. She described fond memories of her family and church guests gathering after dinner for sing-alongs. Verra often felt hungry when she was growing up because her diet consisted of bread and potatoes, but singing and playing the organ seemed to ease her hunger pains and soften the reality of her family's economic status. Verra learned early to lean on the strength of her faith and be grateful for what she did have.

Sitting across from Verra in the retirement community, I couldn't help but notice how her face lit up as she told me how gratifying it was for her to visit nursing homes and lead sing-alongs for residents living in Alzheimer's units. Following Verra's lead, these individuals had no problem remembering songs they'd learned long ago, yet they couldn't remember what they did earlier that same day. Nursing home staffs were baffled by Verra's ability to connect with these people.

Verra could well have been a lonely, bitter old woman because she never married, never had children, and her only living sibling lived far away. Certainly most people purpose their lives around family, so how could Verra's later years be so purposeful without family? Verra's life obviously didn't conform to society's vision of old age. Not only did she make the best of the hand life dealt her, but she was thriving in spite of it! Verra wasn't simply going through the motions of life. No, she did everything with a sense of purpose and love, and it was this sense of purpose—and her perception of the world—that spoke to me the most. Verra believed she made a difference in people's lives, doing work that mattered. She purposed her life around her passion for music, and she was indeed living out what I now call AgePotential.

My encounter with Verra deepened my curiosity to learn more about people like her, and since then, I have been privileged to develop relationships with many "Verras," some of whom you'll meet later on in the book. These thrivers aren't all centenarians, and they don't choose the same exact path, but each one demonstrates how fulfilling and joyful growing old can be. Collectively, these people turned scientific data into reality. Getting to know them and learning their stories made the idea of Generation AgePotential come alive.

Each generation embodies a unique influence and power—and Generation AgePotential is no different. Unlike Gen X, Gen Y, and the Baby Boomers, who were all *born* into their respective generations, anyone from any generation can *choose* to become part of this new generation that lives out what I'm calling Age-Potential. Generation AgePotential is a group of people of mixed ages who are redefining what it means to age by taking ownership of their lives, embracing their chronological age by reimagining their psychological age, seeing a potential to make a difference, and capitalizing on that opportunity. Ultimately, Generation AgePotential validates the ability to *thrive* in later life.

My new concept of AgePotential will shift preexisting negative associations of age. It will align society's thinking with the truths discovered by the latest research on aging and epigenetics. As a visionary gerontologist who studies the process of growing older, I picture aging not as it is commonly depicted today, but as it *could* be. What I am introducing is more than self-help. It's a new way of thinking about what it means to grow older; it's a new vision of aging. And it all starts with your own ability to align your ideas of *aging* with *potential.* Think *aging*, think *potential.* AgePotential is not about aging as much as it is about living—and *living abundantly.* The time has come for us to awaken to the truth that we are all pure potential at every age and stage in life and to acknowledge that we are limited only by the constraints we put on ourselves.

Why isn't everyone already living life with an Age-Potential approach? Most of us are constrained by the stereotypes we've adopted as truths because we have yet to be awakened to the possibilities presented by the latest research. AgePotential is the key difference between *thriving* and merely *surviving* the later years in life. But the potential to thrive starts and ends with you first being awakened! Awareness precedes action. As Gail Sheehy eloquently states, "If every day is an awakening, you will never grow old. You will just keep growing."

Every path to AgePotential is unique. I admire the resolve and ability of the thrivers profiled in this book to live their ordinary lives in such extraordinary ways, defying the status quo. My intention is that their stories and the research presented in the pages that follow will help you find your *own* unique path. My intention is that you will:

Awaken to the power that lies within you to live out your AgePotential.

Awaken to the idea that you were created to live a significant life.

Awaken to the reality that you are the number one influence in your health and aging journey.

Awaken to the fact that nothing holds more power over your body than your thoughts and beliefs.

Awaken to the fact that your genes are your predisposition, not your fate.

Awaken to the mindset that you have a choice in how you age.

Awaken to the new vision of aging.

Awaken to the possibilities beyond the prescribed roles of being a son/daughter, mother/father, grandchild/grandparent, husband/wife, or friend/neighbor.

Awaken to the fact that the way you live your life today will prepare you for tomorrow.

Awaken to the reality that age has potential, age has purpose, age has its advantages. And along with age comes a deeper understanding of self. Aging is a privilege denied to many. Don't regret it. Value it.

Awaken to the invitation set before you: become part of a new generation choosing to live out their AgePotential.

Ultimately, my mission is to educate, empower, and inspire you to live a richer and more independent life by helping you understand the real possibility inherent in our later years. If you open your mind to the ideas and stories that follow, you will experience a genuine **awakening**.

A New Perspective on Aging: Beyond Stereotypes, Socialization, and Fear

What does it mean to age? In other words, how do we, as a society, interpret the physical, mental, and emotional changes we each undergo over time? Contrary to popular belief, "Chronic disease, illness, and disability are not inevitable consequences of aging, but in fact can be prevented or delayed," according to the National Council on Aging's Center for Healthy Aging. This emerging research aligns with my belief that everyone has the ability to achieve his or her AgePotential.

The first step, which is often overlooked, is to address our belief systems around aging. We cannot achieve our potential without consciously realigning our beliefs with the truth and letting go of stereotypes (which are often taken on unconsciously). My concept of AgePotential—a new way of thinking about aging, where people *expect* to live happy, healthy, and fulfilling lives regardless of their age—will be a catalyst for that change.

Let me first address the common perceptions of "old age" among different generations in an effort to show why we may have developed a fear of aging. Generally speaking, people are living longer, and our perceptions of old age shift as we grow older. A recent survey conducted by the Marist Institute for Public Opinion found that Millennials consider old age to start at age sixty-two, Gen-Xers at seventy-one, Baby Boomers at seventy-seven, and individuals in the Greatest Generation at eighty-one. Humans have always had trouble coming to terms with the unknown, and old age is, without a doubt, a much more significant unknown for a Millennial than a Baby Boomer. Nevertheless, it's interesting to note that the survey suggests that the perception of age directly corresponds to a person's chronological age.

So, as you might imagine, reality and perception more closely align as we grow older. Young people, according to Jeffrey Love, research director at AARP, tend to think growing old will be worse than older adults report. Taking the Marist Institute survey and Love's research together, it seems a fear of the unknown and a lack of understanding of how wonderful the aging journey can be strongly influence a person's opinion of what age is "old."

Misconceptions and stereotypes, such as those caused by a lack of understanding, misrepresent the aging process. One common stereotype, for example, depicts older adults as frail and sick. You can imagine how derogatory perspectives like this affect the way older adults feel about their age and stage in life. But aging is not a disease; it is a developmental process. The vast majority of people over sixty-five are healthy enough to engage in most activities of daily living (ADLs), such as bathing, dressing, or preparing meals. And actually, I've met many older thrivers who have the stamina and drive to launch new businesses and nonprofits, run marathons, and more.

Just like thrivers, we can learn to anticipate and adapt to normal age-related changes—such as vision and hearing impairment—and still lead happy, healthy, and active lives. It is wrong to believe that age alone makes us more susceptible to specific diseases or death. Rather, the increased susceptibility comes from neglect or unhealthy habits and a tendency to disengage from the things that keep us youthful—such as dreaming, goal setting, seeking new experiences and learning opportunities, physical activity, making new friendships, and being curious and creative, to name a few. Most people leave these things behind when they move into the second half of life, but keeping them with you is key to maintaining your health and vitality.

We live not only with stereotypes about aging but also with the influence of socialization. Advertisements, the media, and various teachings and observations may be subtle, but they have a profound effect. We are all enmeshed in our early conditioning, for the good and the bad. As a result, many expect the later years to involve the dreaded *D*s of life: disease, decline, depression, denial, dependence, disability, and despair. Without inner work to change this conditioning, most older adults never move beyond "the givens" of aging, which were likely established at a very young age. Bruce Lipton, author of *Biology of Belief*, has found that "our lives are essentially a printout of our subconscious programs, behaviors that were fundamentally acquired from others (our parents, family, and community) before we were six years old."

Thanks to a 2005 study by Szegedy-Maszak, neuroscience also tells us that more than 95 percent of our thoughts and actions originate in the subconscious mind, while less than 5 percent originate in the conscious mind. The control center of the mind, the subconscious, is not governed by reason or thinking but is comprised of habitual, learned responses that often sabotage the conscious mind. Our life aspirations reside in the conscious mind, but our adopted stereotypical beliefs exist subconsciously. They often don't align with the aspirations of the conscious mind. My goal is to *awaken* everyone to these limiting, subconscious beliefs and encourage you to reframe them.

Today, young people are expected to *thrive*, while older adults are expected to merely *survive*. And so it is—what you expect is what you get. The real tragedy is that people come into their later years assuming or expecting the stereotypes will be true, and they then live down to those expectations. In other words, if you think you are "old," that belief will, in time, bring about "older" behavior and lead you to adopt an "older" self-image.

Healthy older adults are all too often socialized into a passive, dependent lifestyle, which requires them to live on someone else's terms (and makes them easier to "manage"). Many young people and older adults alike have fallen into the trap of thinking late life is a time to be "taken care of." Caretakers fall into the trap, too, believing their job is to "take care of" rather than "walk alongside" and empower older adults. What was once a good, protective intention has gradually undermined the real possibility of autonomy and independence in late life, which many older adults are fully capable of. We need to recognize that full health and autonomy are possible at every age, and rather than enable and perpetuate helplessness, we need to take steps toward achieving a healthy lifestyle.

All these negative stereotypes about aging can lead us to fear the aging process, adopt an ageist perspective, or even develop a prejudice against our "feared" future self, as indicated in a 2005 research study by T. D. Nelson. Women around the world seem to worry about aging more than men; however, the specific fears of each sex differ. According to a Bupa Health Pulse study in 2010, the number one fear among women is losing attractiveness or becoming "invisible," and among men, impotence topped the list. Other fears for women—listed in order of importance—include being left alone, financial destitution, cancer, and becoming a burden. Men, on the other hand, fear feeling weaker, becoming irrelevant, losing independence, and losing their minds' full capacity. It's interesting to note that across the board, the fear of losing "what was" overshadows the possibility of "what lies ahead." And what's more, the fact that the survey focuses on what we "fear" in old age, rather than what we "most look forward to," only reinforces the stereotype that there *is* something to fear in old age.

Along that line of thought, could it be that our fear of disease and disability keeps us focused on merely *avoiding* disease instead of *maintaining* health—as if to say, disease is all but inevitable? It's no surprise that dementia was the number one health concern of the twelve thousand male and female Americans surveyed in the 2010 Bupa Health Pulse. Dementia, especially Alzheimer's disease, receives copious media attention, while the potential inherent in late life—and the stories of thrivers, specifically—receives minimal coverage. Without a doubt, this affects society's overall awareness of the possibility to age well, leads to stereotyping, and results in fear.

True, we live in an ageist society that fears growing older and favors youth, yet poll after poll shows that older adults are more content with life, less depressed, and less fearful of death than young people. "I'm a lot more sanguine and comfortable about aging at seventy-six than I was at fifty-six," says George Vaillant, professor of psychiatry at Harvard Medical School and codirector of its Study of Adult Development. Concerns about aging heighten in midlife, which is critical because most people develop their roadmap for late life during that time. It's all the more reason to awaken to your AgePotential early on, so you can avoid living out your future based on unfounded fears. After all, youth is a state of mind, not a number. In mind and body, it is possible to be old at forty and youthful at age eighty.

Thrivers often have a canny way of transcending fear and limitations. For instance, one thriver shared with me that when she is overcome with fear, she recites this acronym: "False Evidence Appearing Real." In their own unique ways, thrivers have learned to replace fear with confidence and love, despite the shortcomings of life and the aging process. Worry is a joy-stealer, and joy is something thrivers have learned to harness. Of course, thrivers have concerns they could worry about, just like the rest of us. But they choose not to. Constant worry and fear eventually leave a person feeling over-whelmed, and according to C. Norman Shealy in *Life Beyond 100: Secrets of the Fountain of Youth,* unresolved fear or worry results in physical illness. Living well and living fully require that we transcend fear.

Not only have thrivers learned to overcome their fears, but they also understand the importance of pres-ent-moment living. Mentally focusing on fear or prob-lems hinders our ability to take action now. Or in other words, allowing the mind to solely focus on a fear can completely disconnect us from what is really happen-ing in the present moment. Present-moment living helps us gain a clear perspective on a given situation as well as develop a rational plan for how to proceed. Of course, it's important to realize that sometimes we can take action and other times we must accept what is out of our control. The following diagram illustrates the process you might go through to gain perspective, because worry, according to Shealy, represents the possibilities more than the probabilities:

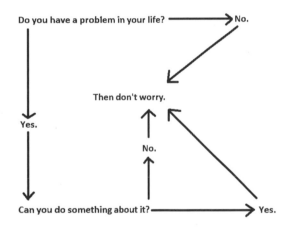

Beyond present-moment thinking and living, older adults may simply have a higher tolerance for uncertainty, and as a result, they are better at coping with fear. According to a study in the *International Journal of Aging and Human Development*, older adults place less value on worrying and have a greater ability to tolerate life's uncertainties than do younger adults. Perhaps our inclination to worry naturally reduces in late adulthood, but I believe we can learn to devalue and detach from worrying at any age. Developing an AgePotential perspective requires us to learn how to take full control of what we can, while letting go of what we can't.

Despite the fact that many older adults have a canny way of coping with fear, are often better able to live in the present moment, and may have a higher tolerance for uncertainty, 50 percent of older adults still do not expect to age well, according to a 2002 report by Sarkisian, Hays, and Mangione. Again, if you expect what you fear the most (which, in many cases, is disease and decline), your fears will become your reality.

Conversely, denying or trivializing the real and positive potential of aging can prevent you from realizing the full spectrum of your talents, intelligence, and emotions. Gene Cohen, MD, PhD, states, "When we come…to expect positive growth with age, such growth can be nurtured." With his book *The Mature Mind*, Cohen teaches us that rich possibilities of life, including the life of the mind, continue well into the latest of our years. We *can* reprogram our thoughts and beliefs to eliminate our fears and work toward achieving our AgePotential. Once you change your beliefs, your experience of aging will change. To positively influence how you age, you only have to be free of fear and believe in yourself and in your ability. In other words, you must simply *expect* to *thrive*—and you will.

Ageism remains subtly, covertly, or unconsciously present, despite the wealth of strong research evidence that suggests older adults are, in fact, mentally and physically capable of living productive lives. The danger lies in the fact that many people still subconsciously take on an ageist perspective without thought, question, reflection, or intentional reframing, and therefore they run the risk of living out a lie.

It is up to each of us as individuals to filter the influences we encounter and decide for ourselves what we will believe about the aging process. I am offering you a new perspective of aging called AgePotential, and with it, you can shed your old perspectives through intentional and conscious effort. Released from overly negative illusions about aging, you will be stirred by new energy, direction, and purpose.

What's more, consciously filtering stereotypical messages will not only help you take a step toward achieving your AgePotential, but it will also keep you from becoming depressed in late life. People who buy into ageist thinking generally slip into some form of depression in late life. And the World Health Organization estimates that by 2020, depression will be the leading cause of "disability-adjusted life years," which means depression will result in years of life lost to "low-grade survival mode" or premature death. Addressing our perceptions and beliefs about aging is clearly a worthwhile effort, since people who have a positive outlook on aging will live on average seven and a half years longer, as reported by a 2008 study by Butler. Another study cited by the Society for Social Work and Research states that older adults who have a positive perception of aging are more likely to have higher self-efficacy and be less depressed. As a result, the medical community should consider perceptions of aging and self-efficacy when developing strategies to prevent and treat depression in older adults.

The best news is that there are so many reasons why we can *expect* to thrive. The human body has a natural ability to adapt and overcome the potentiality of illness and disease, in addition to having remarkable healing powers. We just have to work with our bodies to promote health and vitality. We shouldn't think of aging as a failure of our bodily systems, says Kenneth Minaker, MD, chief of geriatric medicine at Massachusetts General Hospital in Boston and associate professor of medicine at Harvard Medical School.

"Aging is a life-saving process," he says. "It is a process of lifelong adaptation to prevent us from developing cancers that would kill us." The body is naturally self-replenishing; it renews its energies at depletion to return the body to a state of balance. Normal aging is *not* what drains our sustaining energy. Instead, it is our will (or lack thereof) to live life fully that will determine whether our lives become void of meaning and purpose. Indeed there is nothing that leads to rapid premature aging faster than what Stanford physician Walter Bortz calls Disuse Syndrome, a general negligence in attending to one's body and mind.

Despite the prevailing stereotypical perception of old age, society's general attitude toward older adults has steadily improved, which is a direct result of increased education and media attention. For example, the media is enamored with the "Betty White" experience of aging, and it has helped advance a more positive attitude toward older individuals and a better picture of healthy aging. Even though some people attribute Betty's success to her affluence and fame as an actress and comedian, I beg to differ. There are many "Betty Whites" in the world, and I call them thrivers. They are ordinary people living out extraordinary aging experiences. Betty has international visibility, and her story confirms the need for heightened awareness of thrivers in order to advance the possibility of AgePotential. What will tip *you* toward being a thriver—or a non-thriver—is whether you hold the personal belief that the possibility of aging well is a reality for *you*.

To help move us beyond assumption and misconception, I'd also like to discuss the three distinct ways of measuring age. Chronological age is measured by the calendar, psychological age is measured by how old you feel, and biological age is measured in terms of critical life signs and cellular processes. I briefly addressed chronological and psychological ages in the introduction and would now like to touch on biological age.

The biological measurement of age indicates how your cells, tissues, and organs have been affected over time. Biological age is pliable, because lifestyle changes can slow aging at a cellular level. For example, as we age, our telomeres become shorter, and shortened telomeres make people more vulnerable to disease. Telomeres are the ends of chromosomes that serve to protect the genetic DNA from damage. They also act as "cellular clocks" and indicate the age of the cell within the body. Lifestyle changes have been shown to boost telomerase, an enzyme that increases telomere length. Diet, exercise, and a positive mindset can also protect telomeres.

This means healthy habits may slow aging at the cellular level. For instance, a daily routine of exercise over a lifetime can act as a safeguard against the typical effects of biological aging, such as high blood pressure, excess body fat, improper sugar balance, and decreased muscle mass. In contrast, the influence of a negative, self-defeating mindset can indicate that your body's biological age is older than its chronological age. Your body becomes biologically younger or older, depending on your lifestyle habits.

The new science of epigenetics speaks to this. The word *epigenetics* is defined as "control above the genes," or in other words, it means our gene activity is continually modified in response to our life experiences. The concept is antithetical to our traditional understanding of genetic control, the idea that our fate is "dictated" by our genes. Epigenetics suggests you have the power to change the quality of your life by changing your beliefs. *You* can become a thriver.

Another way of putting it, according to Lipton, is that our perceptions of life shape our biology. The single cell's awareness of the environment—not its genes—sets the mechanism of life into motion. The physical and energetic environment of any given cell controls the cell's life. From our cells to our minds, bodies, and spirits, we can choose to perceive ourselves in the context of our environment in different ways, either as perennial victims or as cocreators of our own destinies. And Lipton agrees. He says, "We may act as victims of heredity but we are masters of our own fate." Genes do not dictate our destinies. Nutrition, stress, and emotions can modify genes without changing their basic blueprint.

In other words, we all have predispositions to disease and illness (or "bad" genes), but what deciphers if or when those genes will affect us is a direct result of our thoughts, belief systems, and perceptions of our environments. I have heard this phenomenon described with the analogy of a cell "eavesdropping" on our thoughts. And it's true. Thoughts—the mind's energy—are the catalysts that activate or inhibit the cell.

It's also evident that our biological age does not always reflect our chronological age. What is happening pathologically inside the body may be different than what is presented physically outside the body. Pathogens, or the specific agents causing disease, may lie dormant within the body or be asymptomatic or atypical in nature. In the past, when disease was not physically evident at the time of a person's death, "old age" was an assumed diagnosis. Today, physicians can no longer list "old age" as a cause of death. Instead, they are instructed to list the immediate cause of death and any conditions that led up to it. It is important, therefore, to shed the belief that your increasing chronological age, in and of itself, has a detrimental effect on your biological age.

How empowering is this research with regard to our health and aging journey? Very empowering. According to *Biology of Belief* author Bruce Lipton, "Harnessing the power of your mind can be *more* effective than the drugs you have been programmed to believe you need." Tragically, though, the majority of the population remains unaware of this fact or chooses not to believe it and, as a result, operates on the belief that we are all "victims of our genes." But we aren't. We simply need to rethink the way we age, and in the process of doing so, we need to develop thought patterns that positively affect our cells. Lipton goes on to emphasize that to *fully thrive*, "we must not only eliminate the stressors, but also actively seek joyful, loving, fulfilling lives that stimulate growth processes." In other words, removing life stressors will only do so much—it will only put you in a neutral range of vitality. To be in the positive range of vitality, we must seek positive, fulfilling lives. Again, your biological age directly relates to how you *think* about your mind and body.

Put another way, even though most people associate the adage "use it or lose it" to the body, it can also be applied to the brain. While it was once believed that the brain was hardwired during childhood and there was nothing you could do to change it, today we know the brain is pliable in nature, able to form new cells and neural connections. Neuroscientists often refer to the brain as a malleable, living organ. The term *neuroplasticity* refers to the brain's ability to change in response to new learning and experience.

But as most people age, they tend to fall into routines and avoid opportunities that would engage them in new activities or experiences that could foster neuroplasticity. But it's not enough to fall into routines. You have to learn new things to spur growth of new brain cells—just as thrivers do. According to Janie Clark, MA, president of the American Senior Fitness Association and author of *Brain Fitness for Older Adults*, "We can mitigate the degenerative cognitive loss commonly associated with normal aging by encouraging neuroplasticity." Of course our genes matter, but our thoughts, perceptions of our physical and energetic environments, and lifestyles matter more.

Western medicine has, in the past and to our detriment, failed to acknowledge the mind-body connection. Why is this so alarming? Because, as evidenced by the information I just presented, growing old starts in the *mind*. Since the body follows the mind's lead, the beliefs or vision we hold for our later years is highly important. As Christiane Northrup, MD, states, "Nothing is ever just in your head. Nothing is ever just in your body. They are intrinsically linked—always." The state of the mind is indicative of the state of the body, just as the state of the body is indicative of the state of the mind.

Treating a person as a whole entity—as body, mind, and spirit—is a holistic approach. And a holistic approach to healing goes far beyond simply treating or eliminating symptoms. For example, taking a statin drug for high cholesterol may bring the HDL/LDL measurement within a healthy range, but the real problem—diet, mindset, exercise, or stress—still exists. In holistic medicine, a symptom is considered a message about something that needs attention. So the symptom is used as a guide to look below the surface for the root of the problem. Then what really needs attention can be addressed.

Stress, incidentally, is one of the biggest precursors to disease and premature aging. In a 2008 issue of *Science Daily*, UCLA scientists report that people under chronic stress have shorter telomeres. But thankfully, stress aging is reversible. You can prevent premature aging by learning how to slow down your mind and body. Research by Dean Ornish, MD, shows that life-

style changes and stress management can not only prevent heart disease but may also reverse it. Ornish suggests yoga, meditation, and deep breathing as effective
ways of controlling stress. He also believes that true
motivation for positive, healthy, long-term change
comes not from fear (such as the fear of dying from
a heart attack), but from the desire to feel better and
have a greater zest for life. And his ideas are becoming
more generally accepted. Medicare, the government
health insurance program for Americans age sixty-
five and older, declared the Dean Ornish Program for
Reversing Heart Disease—which advocates a plant-
based and meatless diet, meditation, and regular exercise—the intensive cardiac rehab program in 2010.

Along with stress levels and mindset, nutrition is
another environmental factor that will activate genes
either toward disease and illness or toward prevention
and delay. *The China Study* reports on the most com-
prehensive nutrition study ever conducted. Authors
T. Colin Campbell, PhD, and Thomas M. Campbell
II, MD, state, "Genes do not determine disease on
their own. Genes function only by being activated, or
expressed, and nutrition plays a critical role in determining which genes, good and bad, are expressed." Our
genes are the code to everything in our bodies, good
and bad. However, not all genes are fully expressed all

the time. If they aren't activated, they remain dormant. What determines if a gene is to remain dormant or not is its environment. According to Campbell and Campbell, nutrition (specifically animal protein) is one environmental factor that can turn the bad genes on or off.

While modern medicine *is* doing a good job of phasing out premature death, it cannot assure a high quality of life. Only you can do that for yourself, as the research suggests. Again, the majority of illnesses and premature deaths can be traced back to lifestyle choices. There are well known dangers, for instance, connected to drugs, alcohol, nicotine, and unprotected sexual activity. Less recognized dangers include the impact of excess sugar, caffeine, negativity, and the like. Combined with deficiencies in exercise, nutritious foods, and self-esteem, these lifestyle choices gradually accumulate and can have harmful effects. With time, they diminish the quality of the "environment" within us and can set the stage for illness. Quality of life—both in the present and in the future—is actually determined by the many seemingly unimportant choices you make every day.

For those who really want to live healthy, independent lives into old age, the research presented thus far provides a roadmap. Environmental factors such as stress, nutrition, exercise, thoughts, and belief systems are all things we can control and influence. This is empowering. We no longer have to think or believe we are victims of our genes. The research clearly indicates what is possible—with your lifestyle and mindset, you can dictate how your genes are going to play out. We should no longer expect the stereotypes of aging, but expect to thrive instead.

In sum, and according to Harvard psychologist George Vaillant, aging is a learned process. In other words, if you learned or adopted the old paradigm of aging—the belief that the power to age well lies in external factors such as genes, medicine, doctors, or circumstances—you can *unlearn* it. American writer and futurist Alvin Toffler claims that the "illiterate" of the future are not those who cannot read or write, but those who are unwilling to learn, unlearn, and relearn. Aging with vitality is an acquired perspective. We are what we repeatedly do. Healthy aging, therefore, is not an act, but a habit. A lifestyle. A mindset. A choice. The good news is that there is so much to be learned and developed. Again, it's up to each of us to shape the way we live and age.

Even though the subtleties of stereotypes, socialization, and fear continue to shape the general perception of old age, presently there is more and more research supporting alternative perspectives. And as individual awareness heightens and expands, the collective awareness will shift. Remember, the possibility for all of us to reach our AgePotential is real, but AgePotential is not a collective experience. Instead, it requires individual choice and intention. Society as a whole may still cling to the old paradigm of aging, but that doesn't mean you have to. Herein lies your power. If there is one concept I hope you will understand and believe, it's that *you* are the number one influence on your aging journey. But you must believe it to be true.

A Winning Equation for Thriving in Later Life

Age (life experience & wisdom) + Potential (possibility in waiting) = AgePotential

AgePotential + Awareness + Action = Thriver

What Is AgePotential?

AgePotential is a concept I coined with the intention of shifting our collective awareness and association of age to potential. Think *aging*, think *potential*. Most people attribute potential to youth, but potential is not defined or limited by age. We are pure potential at every age and stage of life. Reframe your aging vision to AgePotential and begin living your best life.

Living out your potential in old age does not necessarily mean to be without disease or disability. However, the term *thrivers* is often used to describe individuals of advanced age who continue to live out their potential, be engaged, and contribute extensively by using their talents, gifts, and energies to the betterment of themselves and others. But AgePotential is not a comparison of people and their aging process; therefore, it does not imply that one individual ages better or worse than others or that an individual has to reach a set of imposed criteria that does not include subjective health and personal biography. Rather, AgePotential reflects the individual ability to overcome and adapt to life's trials and tribulations in order to reach the highest potential, while accounting for health status and life circumstances.

AgePotential is a realization that each of us can continue to evolve throughout our lifespans and then act on that realization with courage. Your potential is not quite a *thing*, but it is more than just an *idea*. It lies in a latent state between idea and reality, where all things are possible but have yet to be developed. AgePotential can be cultivated—innate talents and skills are lying dormant within you and me, waiting to be awakened and developed.

You may wonder why we aren't already fulfilling our AgePotential. Common barriers to living out AgePotential stem from socialization and stereotypes, as discussed earlier in the book, and they may include an ageist belief system, relinquishment of power, fear, lack of present-day purpose and meaning, an inability to live in the present, or the limited visibility of positive aging role models. The fundamental barrier to achieving AgePotential, however, seems to be the simple fact that most people do not believe in themselves or their ability to be their own best advocates.

Living out AgePotential is really about devoting yourself to creating something that gives you purpose and meaning. Developing "self" is not a goal; it is a process—a lifetime process. Life is a continuum, a continuous series of change and shifts with no "arrival," per se. To be alive means to be in a constant state of change. And to be *fully* alive means to embrace the change. Change is inevitable; growth is optional. Our tendency to want to "coast through" our later years is extremely detrimental to the natural ebb and flow of life. Resistance to change is, in essence, resistance to the flow of life.

A single change can create a habit of momentum. Nobody can go back to the time of birth to start over, but anyone can initiate a new way of thinking or make a "new beginning" today in order to create a "new ending." Today is the day to unleash your potential and express your uniqueness by committing to all you are intended to be.

AgePotential is *not* a means of striving for acceptance or validation. Our inherent value comes from within, not from external validation. Instead, AgePotential is about bearing out all you were created for and intended to be. I believe we all have aging potential—the key is to access it. You are here for a reason, no matter whether you are forty, sixty, or eighty years of age. You make a difference. To embrace AgePotential is to embody the belief that some of the best days of your life are yet to happen and to be inspired to push onward and upward toward where you haven't been. Each time you look deeper into yourself, you find incredibly beautiful treasures waiting to be discovered. Remember, you were created in the image of the Divine. Motivational speaker Lou Holtz says, "I can't believe that God put us on this earth to be ordinary." AgePotential is a path leading to the extraordinary within each of us.

AgePotential Principles

AgePotential is unique to each person, yet there are some common, core ideals that set thrivers apart. These ideals can be learned, which makes the possibility of becoming a thriver available to everyone. Truth is transferable. Knowledge becomes powerful only when it is applied. So herein lies your power to become a thriver. Consider these principles and apply them to your life.

Demonstrate Personal Responsibility

Stepping up to claim personal responsibility for your life involves extreme courage at any age, but the reward of an independent, self-directed life is empowering. In the field of gerontology, we refer to a model of personal responsibility called "new gerontology," first introduced by M. B. Holstein and M. Minkler in 2003. New gerontology is based on the idea that we can participate actively in our own lives, and it promotes prevention. Its goal is to help you modify individual behaviors throughout your life in order to avoid decrements and losses that result from neglect and/or abuse of the mind, body, and spirit.

In fact, new gerontology reflects the sentiment of people all over the world. One of the findings of the Bupa Health Pulse report—which includes research findings based on the participation of more than thirteen thousand individuals in twelve countries—is that "the majority of respondents in 7 out of 12 countries surveyed think it is the responsibility of each individual to ensure that they keep well." The survey results align and support the personal responsibility principle of AgePotential. I have observed that thrivers are self-initiators and have no problem being accountable for their lives. In fact, personal responsibility empowers them to be the captains of their own ships.

So how important are lifestyle choices? Jan Maurer, MD, vice president and medical director at Health Dialog, puts it quite bluntly: "Americans need a wake-up call. People need to realize that lifestyle factors are actually life-and-death factors." The problem most people have is that they want things to stay the same—but also to get better. People are living longer, and they desire for these extra years to be healthy and full of vitality. Since our health status directly affects our quality of life, when people neglect to make healthy lifestyle choices, it undermines the overall health and quality of life they say they want. Over time, our minds, bodies, and spirits need more attention in order to maintain basic well-being. The disconnect I have observed is in what people want and what they are willing to do or not do. Ironically, people want to be "in control," but then they continually relinquish the control they *do* have through poor lifestyle choices and negative or ageist mindsets toward their health and aging journey.

People unknowingly give their power away when they resign themselves to the belief that the power to age well lies outside themselves—in their genes, their doctors, their medications, or in their circumstances. *The real power, however, lies within the level of awareness and our unique perceptions, beliefs, and choices.* The number one influence on how you age is *you*! Thrivers understand the benefits of taking ownership for their health and aging journeys—and because of that awareness, they willingly accept the personal responsibility.

As you might or might not have deduced, the real cause of premature death is often directly related to individual choice and behavior. This fact alone should clarify the importance of personal responsibility as it relates to health. Over 75 percent of healthcare spending goes to preventable conditions, or illnesses that people cause with their own behavior. If we want to "fix" healthcare, why not start by putting energy into our own health as a prevention mechanism? Personal responsibility and self-control are clear trademarks of AgePotential and bring a person to think, "If it's going to be, it's up to me."

I guarantee that the best day of your life is the one on which you decide your life is your own. Your life really begins the day you step into your own voice and power to live your best life. People who live out their AgePotential inevitably want to be in the driver's seat of their life and exert their power of choice and control. Leadership expert John C. Maxwell points out, "Successful and unsuccessful people do not vary greatly in their abilities. They vary in their desire to reach their potential." Is it your desire to live and age to your potential? If so, then you must be willing to take responsibility for your life.

Question Limited Thinking

Thrivers are conscious creators of their lives, not mind-less acceptors. They recognize what the stereotypes, socialization, and fear around aging really are: limited beliefs based on fear. Transformation is often more about unlearning than learning. The first step toward aging to your potential is to challenge your belief system, for nothing holds more power over the body than beliefs of the mind. Byron Katie, creator of "The Work" program, emphasizes how "an unquestioned mind is the world of suffering." She goes on to explain, "*I discovered that when I believed my thoughts, I suffered, but that when I didn't believe them, I didn't suffer, and that this is true for every human being. Freedom is as simple as that. I found that suffering is optional. I found a joy within me that has never disappeared, not for a single moment. That joy is in everyone, always.*" Most of what we normally think, say, and do is habitual. The mind is a perfect servant, as it will do whatever it is told. The idle mind, the mind left to atrophy, is at risk of resigning to the socialized belief of inevitable decline.

So what are beliefs, and how will they affect our aging process? I am not referring to mere positive thinking. To transform your thinking, you must *believe* a new thought to be true on *both* an emotional and intellectual level. Simply believing in something intellectually isn't enough. Take this statement, for example: "As I grow older, I will become frail and dependent." Intellectually, you may know this is not true, but emotionally, you may still believe it. Rational or not, beliefs determine our thoughts, feelings, and behaviors. While empowering beliefs can support us en route to our greatest potential, limiting beliefs do not serve us. Instead, they hinder us from pursuing our dreams and living fully to our potential. You can now unleash your life by addressing the limiting beliefs you hold.

Just as a body cleanse helps maintain or restore physical health, a "mind cleanse," cleansing ourselves of limiting beliefs, is imperative to maintaining our mental health. We need to reflect in order to become aware of our limiting beliefs. Reflection is simply looking *within* so you can look *out* with a broader, yet more accurate, perspective. Identifying our subconscious limiting beliefs initiates a change or shift in our minds. It allows us to adopt new conscious beliefs that will enhance our present-day lives, not limit them.

The purpose of identifying a limiting belief is to replace it with a new belief that does not limit. Christiane Northrup recommends this: "Rather than think you need to go on an archaeological dig into your personal history, just look at your life in the present moment to see what your past beliefs have created." It is not necessary to understand, fix, or change the past before you can begin aging mindfully.

Recognizing what holds us back is the first step to releasing it. But truly ridding your mind of old thoughts and beliefs that do not serve you now involves putting energy into developing *new* thoughts and beliefs. That is, if you put thought-energy toward nothing more than ending an undesirable thought or pattern, you will only perpetuate it. It is better to dedicate your thought-energy toward creating new desired outcomes. The old views will eventually atrophy and die once they no longer receive thought-energy.

Here's how to identify a limiting belief:

1. **Listen to your self-talk.**

   What is your inner voice telling you? Do you find yourself saying such things as these?

   "I'm too old to do that."

   "I used to do that when I was young."

   "If I were younger, I would be more apt to try that."

2. **Understand your attitude about aging.**

Do you believe you can lead a fulfilling and robust life, regardless of age?

Do you know you are the number one influence in how you age?

Do you dread growing older?

Do you despise birthdays?

Are you driven by fear?

3. **Pay attention to current circumstances.**

When we're not happy with our circumstances in life—our careers, our relationships, our lifestyles—it often indicates there's a self-sabotaging limiting belief under the surface. If you aren't moving toward what you want in life, chances are, an unconscious limiting belief is tripping you up.

In "The Work," a method of self-inquiry, Katie suggests this approach:

1. Write down a limiting belief.
2. Ask, "Is this true?"
3. Ask, "Am I 100% sure it's true?"
4. What is this limiting belief doing to me?
5. Who would I be without this limiting belief?
6. Reframe the belief.

The journey of conscious living requires constant inquiry into what is true and real. It is not a path of following what is popular or acceptable. Thinking for oneself has become a lost art; few people resist the pressure to "fit in."

But there comes a time when each of us must examine for ourselves what we believe in and why. Age is not a limitation, unless we allow it to be. I encourage people to go on a radical diet. No, not a food diet, but a "thought diet." I want you to abstain from allowing yourself to use your *age* as an excuse or a limitation. Your potential to contribute, create, and innovate exists within you for your entire life. Since our thoughts and perceptions affect us down to a cellular level (which, again, is the premise of epigenetics), it is vital that we consciously align our thinking of the aging process to the potentiality that exists within us all. We will be unable to do so, however, until we are first made aware of that potentiality.

In summary, your life is what your thoughts make it. The way you take in information, either mindfully or mindlessly, determines how you will use it later. We are surrounded every day by subtle—and not-so-subtle—signals that aging is an undesirable period of decline. These signals make it difficult throughout adulthood to continue developing a healthy mindset toward aging. But once we shake the negative clichés that dominate our thinking, we can mindfully open ourselves to the possibilities of a productive life, no matter how old we are.

Cultivate a Mindful, Proactive Approach
Mindfulness is all about intentional living; in other words, mindfulness is living your life on purpose with a conviction and openness to keep evolving as a person. Mindlessness, on the other hand, is a life of habit "just because" you have always been or lived this way. Choosing a familiar course results in mental laziness, rigidity, and a lack of growth and personal development.

Just as mindlessness is the rigid reliance on old ways, mindfulness is the continual creation of new ones. When we are mindful, we *see* choices and options that generate new endpoints. Mindfulness implies open-ness to new information, which is vital to AgePotential. This openness spurs imagination and creativity, as well as new energy. People who embody mindfulness are masters at reframing the context of a situation (often a challenge, problem, or limitation) to better serve them-selves. The process of reframing allows us to shift our negative view of a constraining situation into a posi-tive view of a situation full of potential, regardless of whether the experience ultimately changes. Reframing is a quintessential skill of any thriver. Reframed per-ceptions are a great source of hope and empowerment.

New ways of thinking lend themselves to new ways of being and becoming. Becoming the person you are meant to be involves allowing all that is meant for you to flow into your life. That often involves change. In fact, since life is nothing but a series of shifts and changes, our aging process will inevitably involve change and adaptation. Why should that surprise us?

There may be a need to check in with how you have viewed change in the past. How have you adapted to life's interruptions and transitions so far? You may need to reframe how you view change, so you can begin to embrace all that change has to offer. What appears as an ending may be best viewed as a wonder-ful new beginning.

Our ability to change is directly related to our awareness—the greatest agent for change. And awareness, our open-mindedness, is essential to living out AgePotential. Your life is an expression of your own level of awareness. What you become is the result of what you do today. The way you live your life today is preparing you for tomorrow. Today is the youth of your old age.

Now that we understand what it means to be mindful and open to change, we have to learn to fully embrace that attitude through proactivity. Being proactive means you plan ahead and take action to ward off the possible hindrances of life—and you establish a goal to maintain your sense of purpose, health, and youthful vibrancy. On the contrary, being reactive means that you wait to react *after* life events or transitions, such as illness, occur. They may take you by surprise.

The most significant effect of proactivity, however, is that it invites us to contemplate the future. Envisioning a compelling future leads the body to where you want it to go. Neglecting to envision your future keeps you from developing the intentional direction your body needs to thrive.

Consider this an example of being reactive: Are you waiting until you are "older" to think or plan for the second half of your life? We have been socialized not to think about growing older, but denial and avoidance do not make reality go away. In fact, such avoidance will inevitably lead to illness and depression—and a "survivalist" approach to aging. Don't be fooled into thinking you are "set" for later life just because you have your end-of-life directives or nursing home insurance. While these actions may prove to be valuable, if they are your only proactive steps, you are in essence planning only to "survive" later life.

May I suggest you put your thought-energy and time into planning a life that empowers you to stay healthy and purposeful? In other words, make plans for *living*, not for *dying*. Being a proactive thinker is key to achieving AgePotential. Thrivers tend to ask themselves questions such as, "How do I intend to live the second half of my life? What does growing old mean to me? What do I believe about my ability and capability to continue engaging and contributing all throughout my life? Do I consider myself to be the creative force in my aging journey? How do I intend to keep living my life with meaning and purpose? Do I have a vision of myself living to be age seventy, eighty, ninety, and beyond?"

As you can see, being mindful and proactive requires action and commitment—yet equally important is the ability to allow things to unfold as they are meant to. Being in the flow of life means being flexible and open to recognizing the treasures life is offering, even when the package doesn't look as we imagined it would. Being "in the flow" requires us to discern between exerting control and adapting to the inevitable loss of control in our lives. We must learn to observe the role control plays in our lives—to adopt the attitude that everything will turn out as planned, rather than to obsess over an outcome that may or may not be under our control. Those who embrace AgePotential choose to focus on what they can do rather than what they cannot do. And by accepting life as it is, they also achieve peacefulness and contentment.

A lack of flexibility, on the other hand, often keeps some of the best ideas and opportunities from being discovered. If we are rigid, we tend to become "set in our ways," which makes the second half of our lives highly limited. This is where the power of proactivity and awareness comes in. Awareness can produce unlimited change. *You* have the power—and the choice—to avoid becoming rigid and closed-minded. If you are open and if you expect the best in life, you will receive the best of life.

It's imperative to note that AgePotential embodies maverick-type thinking. Research indicates that

70 percent of people who watch television are not watching something they are interested in; instead, they watch for the sake of watching. Unfortunately, many people run their whole lives that way—passive and indifferent. Maverick thinkers, on the other hand, are people who think for themselves. Our goal in life should not be to meld into the crowd, but to be authentic to ourselves. It's no easy task, since conformity is one of society's most difficult forces to escape. But maverick thinkers have an inherent belief that their lives matter, that they can make a difference and have a positive impact. They would encourage you to believe in your own cause, follow your truth, and stick to your journey, even if you have to walk the path on your own. The AgePotential approach is not one-size-fits-all; it is unique to you. Thrivers understand this, and their lives reflect their unique talents, values, and passions.

As you consider how to shape a mindful, proactive approach to your aging journey, keep in mind that the body is an expression of the mind. If you want a healthy, robust, functional body, then your thoughts and beliefs must sustain that quality of life. Again, be in tune to your inner dialogue. Be mindful of how you are presently living, because this is a direct indicator of what late life will hold for you. Remember, mindfulness can be developed over time. There is a tendency to think of aging as a "future" life experience, but in reality, we are all aging every day. So baby steps of change now will, over time, lead to real change. Never lose sight of your vision, your goals, and your passions. Gary Lew's famous quote reminds us, "This is your world. Shape it or someone else will."

Create a Passion-Centered Life

Health is more than just the absence of disease; it is the presence of vitality. And vitality of the mind and spirit is as important as vitality of the body. As the body cannot live without food, so the soul cannot live without meaning and passion. Using your gifts and talents brings purpose and fulfillment to your day and your life. Passion often evolves out of a deep concern about something important to you, and it propels you to act on that concern. Passion gives wings to your ideas. Passion means believing you can make a difference. Passion drives you beyond yourself and your inner circle to act on behalf of the greater good.

Following what makes you naturally curious will lead you to unleash your potential. With age, we become more discerning of our time and become more focused on what truly matters in life. The purpose of a job is to make a living, not to make a life; likewise, retirement means retiring from a job, but it does not mean retiring from life. Unfortunately, we aren't encouraged to keep dreaming and evolving in retirement. But AgePotential is all about doing what other people only talk or think about doing.

It may feel countercultural to develop and follow your passions, and in many ways, it is—especially as you age. The reward comes in knowing you can continue to grow and use your talents, gifts, and time for a greater good—even, or especially, after retirement. Thrivers don't let someone who gave up on his or her dreams talk them out of going after theirs. They intentionally surround themselves with people who support them in their quests to fulfill their dreams. Do you have an inspiring peer group with equally lofty ideals and goals? Thrivers make it their goal to grow, in some way, every day.

The best news is that passion does not deplete you—it energizes you. It affects every aspect of your life by becoming a driving force and replacing dread and fear and complacency with action. What's more, it doesn't have to be some high-profile kind of thing. It's unique to you. It's your gift, and we all have one. For example, Fred from the book *The Fred Factor* is a postman who is an ordinary person living an ordinary life in an extraordinary way. The "Freds" of the world are not motivated by recognition or reward but have a genuine desire to be the *best* they can be. Fred ultimately got the world's attention by going beyond the "expected" and making his best effort with a joyful attitude to give exceptional service as a postman. Mark Sanborn, author of *The Fred Factor*, was fortunate enough to be on Fred's delivery route.

Just as Fred *chose* not to believe he needed a certain "position" in life to make a difference, so too are the people who live out AgePotential. They know better than to think only young people can live significant lives. The ability to make a significant difference is not limited by age, life position, or circumstance. Similarly, an extraordinary life and aging experience does not require affluence. Purpose, passion, and meaning are accessible to all. Mark Sanborn says, "Nobody can prevent you from choosing to be exceptional." It comes down to how you *choose* to approach your life and aging journey. The potential of age is the opportunity to carry the Fred philosophy into your later years and to make every moment, day, year, and decade a significant one. You have the power, the choice, and the control to be who you want to be and make the impact you want to make.

When a person is driven by passion, that energy spills over into all aspects of life. It becomes a wellspring. Since passion is so invigorating and provides a sense of purpose and meaning, you may wonder why more people don't choose to cultivate it. After all, passionate people are generally more joyful. Usually, complacency and an unwillingness to move outside our comfort zones keep us from deviating from the familiar. It takes real courage to embrace passion. I've heard people say we have been socialized into being ordinary; but people like Fred and Verra, whom I discussed in the introduction, challenge that limited way of thinking. AgePotential is a path leading to the extraordinary within each of us. We are all born with a great capacity to make a significant difference—and minimizing that reality is detrimental to ourselves and the world.

Now that you understand the importance of passion, may I challenge you to entertain the thought of creating change? Take, for example, Terry Hitchcock's compassion for single parents. At age fifty-seven, Terry ran the equivalent of seventy-five marathons in seventy-five consecutive days. As his website states, "He travelled over 2,000 miles to bring awareness to the financial and emotional hardships faced by single parents and their children—everyday heroes who run quiet, yet extraordinary daily marathons."

Terry proved that *impossible* is only a word. "I firmly believe human beings can accomplish anything they put their minds to. All they need to get started is someone to show them it's possible," says Terry. The passion that drove Terry to action exists within us all. Through example, he encourages us all to take that first step of turning passion into action: "Everybody is looking for a reason to continue, a reason to believe in themselves, and I just use [my run] as an example that, hey, if I can do this crazy thing, you can achieve your dream."

And dreams and passion come in all forms. In 2008, Julia Immonen watched a video on human trafficking that forever changed her life. Instead of merely feeling empathetic, Julia chose to bring a greater *awareness* to this injustice. Her passion fueled her and four other women to row the Atlantic for forty-five days to raise awareness about this issue.

But when Julia came up with the idea to row across the Atlantic, she had a few challenges to overcome: She had to find team members who could train and spend forty-five days at sea. With a full-time job, Julia herself had little time for training. And most importantly, she had never spent *any* time at sea—or ever sailed or rowed, for that matter. But the one thing that kept her afloat was her passion for fighting the growing problem of human trafficking.

I include Terry's and Julia's passion stories to heighten your *awareness* of what is possible when the willingness to act on an idea is combined with passion. Passion has the power to turn the ordinary into the extraordinary. What do Terry, Julia, Fred, and Verra have in common? They are common people doing common things uncommonly well. They are all acting on their passions. This is something we can do at any age.

In sum, thrivers are inspired by their passions and have a keen sense of who they are and what they are capable of being. They tend not to settle for less. Imagine what the world would be like if everyone identified their passions and talents and acted on them—especially during their later years, when so many people tend to waste away in complacency. What a world it could be. I believe we were all born with an innate uniqueness waiting to be discovered and used for the greater good. Believe that your life matters, because it truly does. And believe that you can make a difference, because you will.

In conclusion, it is my belief that our capacity to contribute and live fully—to thrive—is not based on age but on the willingness to believe we *can* thrive. Then, we must choose to act on that belief. I want to show you that this type of aging experience requires you to demonstrate personal responsibility; question limited thinking; cultivate a mindful, proactive approach; and create a passion-centered life.

Remember, the more you grow as a person, the more you have to share with the world. When we discover new dimensions of ourselves—just like the thrivers you will soon meet in the next section—we can discover our true passions. This ability to embrace change reignites the spark for life and ultimately puts life back into our steps, helping us achieve our AgePotential.

Thriver Profiles

In a world teeming with ageist stereotypes and beliefs, it is important to seek out positive, real-life role models who prove there is unlimited potential in aging. The following profiles feature ten thrivers living extraordinary lives well into their later years. They share their stories in their own words. Their ages span a number of decades, the youngest "forever at thirty-nine." One thriver still claims to be an ageless "thirty-nine," proving that how we think shapes who we are.

As you will see, these thrivers are just like you and me. They come from all walks of life and have experienced a full spectrum of ups and downs. Their stories are meant to inspire and illustrate the potential to live full, purposeful lives at any age.

After each thriver profile, I include brief commentary to bridge each story to the concepts outlined earlier in this book. I focus on one key aspect from each thriver's story, although there are many common traits running throughout all ten profiles. My hope is that the insight you gain from each thriver story motivates and propels you to begin to take small steps that lead you toward your own unique path of AgePotential.

Milt "Beaver" Adams
Age 84

Let me tell you a story.

New Year's Eve, 1969. I sat down on the davenport in our Edina, Minnesota, home, two champagne flutes in my left hand, a fizzing bottle of champagne in my right. My wife, Jean, played with a strand of pearls around her neck, her worries causing her to fidget, as she often did. I poured some of the sparkling drink for each of us. "Here's to our new beginning in 1970," I said, our glasses meeting with a *clink*.

"Beaver, what are we going to do for money?" Jean said.

There it was, the fearful question I knew had been on her mind all day—the date of December 31, 1969. It was the day I left my fifteen-year career in corporate America to seek my own adventures in the business world; it was the day I made the first step in self-employment that would carry me and my family through the rest of our days.

We had three kids, two car payments, a mortgage, and five hundred dollars in the bank. Most of my close peers likely viewed me as a fool, though a few might have been envious. My own emotions were also mixed—excitement, dread, anxiety, and eagerness all pulled me forward. At the heart of my decision was a desire for fulfillment—but I didn't have an obvious next step. I didn't know when my next paycheck would be arriving or in what amount it would be or from where it would come. What *would* we do for money? I truly didn't know.

What I did know was that I would eventually find my next step and my family would be okay. I knew I could control my own destiny, and I could be my own boss, in control of my own future. I wanted more than a salary; I wanted true passion. Whatever the next step would be, I knew it would be exhilarating. As I looked over at Jean, I grabbed her free hand.

"I don't know, Jean," I said, "and furthermore, I don't care."

I was born on June 17, 1928. My story really starts on a sad note, when I was four years old. It was ten o'clock in the morning, and my father was out on an errand to pick up Grandma's cookies for a picnic we were to have later (her cookies were famous in my family—delicious, but hard as rocks the next day). I have been told I was my father's shadow, always trailing behind him wherever he went. On most occasions,

I would have joined him on such an excursion, but this time it was decided I would stay back for a reason I don't quite remember. It was on this errand that his small Ford Model T was hit by a large, fancy touring rig. His car wrapped around a tree, and he died later that day. I have very few memories of my father—I certainly can't remember his voice. However, I have a clear memory of my very pregnant mother sitting on the edge of the bed with tears streaming down her face.

The woman driving the other vehicle belonged to a very prominent family in town, and she was drunk that morning. In later years, I contemplated knocking on the woman's door to introduce myself, but each time the thought crossed my mind, I thought better of it. At the point I considered confronting her, she was elderly—what if my confrontation gave her a heart attack? I didn't want her death to weigh on my conscience like my father's death probably did on hers.

After my father died, my mother, along with me and my two kid sisters, moved in with my maternal grandparents, Henry and Hannah. A few years later, my mother succumbed to illness, and she died as well. By the time I was nine years old, I was an orphan.

From that point on, I was raised by my grandparents. Being an orphan was a key influence in the development of my personality; living with my grandparents and my teenage aunts and uncles, I was now one of nine in the household. I was nicknamed "Beaver"—partially for my buckteeth, partially for my overly busy nature. The name stuck. I liked it because it made me different from the rest.

Even as a child, I got my energy through talking with people, learning their stories, and sharing my stories with them. It was hard to get noticed among six other kids, all vying for attention, so I earned a reputation for being hyperactive (which my schoolteachers confirmed with exasperation). Later in life, I discovered I had ADHD as a child, as well as in adulthood. Today, a child with ADHD is put on drugs and subdued. Back then, I was simply called a "hellion" or "holy terror." As a child, my ADHD, coupled with my longing for attention and love from people, made me a bit of a nightmare for my teachers. I was in the principal's office every day. They even moved me up a grade, just to get rid of me.

I now look at that combination—being an orphan with ADHD—as a gift. It's an idiosyncrasy that has allowed me to bring people together. Part of that gift is that I am able to recognize idiosyncrasies in others as well; I can see what makes their stories unique. I can make connections happen for people—synapses that make me feel good because they make other people feel good. It's what made me feel good about my choice to enter the world of self-employment at a time in American history when working forty-five years for one corporation and then retiring was what everyone planned and hoped for. But I recognized that my ability to be my fullest self—to bring in as much love and make as many connections as I could—would never be realized if I was fitting into the box defined by someone else.

The great thing about the world today is that it is ripe for entrepreneurship. A person of any age can make a living by being himself or herself. As I changed and grew older, so did my work because it was never anything outside of whom I was. In our culture, we invest so much time in our careers—93,600 hours, to be exact, if we're talking a forty-five-year career at forty hours per week. If we don't feel like our true, full selves in our work, it means we're not living authentically. I'm not suggesting everyone must become an entrepreneur. It's about writing your own story in your work. When you recognize your own gifts, you can identify the career path that will allow those gifts to blossom. Your gifts might not be viewed as gifts by everyone you encounter; some might view them as weaknesses. But you have the choice to know better.

In 1998, after twenty-eight years of doing different

forms of advertising, marketing, and development for different companies—from working a marketing job for Billy Graham's film division to developing a system for consumers to be informed about their dental health practitioners—I rededicated myself to the down-to-earth kind of storytelling I always loved exploring. I did this through publishing books. Named after the moniker given to me more than sixty years earlier, Beaver's Pond Press became my greatest vocation.

At Beaver's Pond Press, where my ever-evolving career has taken me, I spend my days with authors who need me to recognize their gifts and help them use those gifts creatively. I listen to their ideas, help their ideas blossom into better ideas, and figure out how to see those ideas to fruition. I help them be their full, true selves as they tell their stories through their best books possible. Stories are the links that tie us all together—the links that tie the entire world together. For me and my true self, there's no greater way to bring people together than to help their stories live forever in books.

I discovered early in my life that fulfillment doesn't have a beginning nor does it have an end. It's not granted by social standards of success. A car. A title. A house. These are things people use to judge your success, as well as their own success. However, these things all mean something different to each person, and that's why these measurements aren't real. The only measurement of fulfillment you can count on is your *own*, based on how you feel about the job you have done and how you have helped.

You know you're successful and fulfilled if you feel complete in your own skin. If you feel in control of your own destiny. If you're passionate and excited about what you're doing, and yet you're still looking for ways to grow. True fulfillment doesn't come from arriving; rather, it comes from infinite growth and allowing yourself to live without bounds at every age.

Being fulfilled has to be an evolving process. I ask myself at every new stage of life: *Am I being fulfilled? If not, why not? How should I keep evolving?* I realize that to be always fulfilled, I need to always evolve, based on my new circumstances and options, and always create new goals. As evidence of this final point, whenever my old friends see me, they ask, "Beaver, what are you doing now?"

....

Risk Taking...

According to *Webster's Dictionary*, to *thrive* means to grow vigorously, to flourish. For Milt, embracing the unknown and letting go of the comforts of a stable job were risks he needed to take in order to grow into the person he felt called to be. Take note: with this choice, Milt was swimming upstream, as this was "at a time in American history when working forty-five years for one corporation and then retiring was what everyone planned and hoped for."

Learning to take calculated risks improves our self-confidence and ability to manage whatever life deals us. In a world where certainty is rare, this type of inner strength can be the difference between flourishing and floundering. I often hear people describe how unhappy, bored, unchallenged, and burned out they feel, but they never deviate from the familiar path. Why? Could it be the risk factor? Taking a risk is taking a leap of faith. There is no guarantee that everything will work out exactly how you anticipate. But Milt would attest that you experience many benefits simply from trying something new.

What is your attitude toward taking risks? Think back to a time when you chose—or were forced—to stretch yourself or your thinking. I bet you felt outside of your comfort zone. To let go of the familiar is a courageous act.

To become your best self requires making decisions that lead to action. You will never have enough information to make the perfect decision, but life is about making decisions based on the information you do have. There are no crystal ball guarantees. We must accept that there's an element of risk with most decisions we make. And bear in mind that deciding *not* to move forward or take a risk is still making a decision to stick with the status quo, to put up with the circumstances you're currently in.

Thrivers are willing—at least occasionally—to make bold moves, to take intelligent gambles. They knowingly accept that every venture involves some risk. They weigh the pros and cons, plan for the worst, and hope for the best. And you can, too. For Milt, the risk of the temporary financial insecurity was worth taking, because he was leaving the corporate world to pursue his dreams. In Milt's words, "I wanted more than a salary; I wanted true passion." He wanted to do work that held significance and meaning for him.

After making the change, Milt enabled himself to become the captain of his own ship, doing what he loved. And more importantly, he helped others tell their stories and spread their own messages through published books. Passion drove Milt to taking that initial step, that risk. His story shows how by taking risks in an effort to pursue our passions, we can achieve anything we set our minds to.

From my experience in working with thrivers, I see

they are most willing to take risks required for achieving an authentic life. This approach to life is not driven by egotism, but by a desire to feel alive and to make an impact on the world. Milt's innermost desire may have been what Harry Emerson Fosdick alludes to in this quote: "Life is like a library owned by the author. In it are a few books which he wrote himself, but most of them were written for him." So many of our thoughts and actions are influenced by other people's thoughts, values, and desires. But Milt wanted to be authentic, to write and live his own story, and to help others do the same.

Milt's story challenges us to take risks that will help us become our best selves. What risk will you take today, tomorrow, or next month to start living your best life? When will you, like Milt, start writing your own story—knowing that both you and the world will be better for it?

Lynette Crane

Age 75

From a very young age, I assumed I was going to live a long time and I needed to take care of myself in order to be in good shape for all the adventures life would bring me.

I had models of resilient people in my life: as a young ballet dancer, I noted how fit and lively my teachers were. My first teacher was a slim and beautiful woman, then middle-aged, who dressed in a leotard, tights, and ballet slippers. She demonstrated steps for us, doing them more beautifully than we youngsters could. She died at the age of ninety-six, still slim and beautiful.

Why did she die? Her heart and lungs were strong, as was her whole body. She simply decided that because all her contemporaries, including her husband, were gone, it was time for her to go. With her iron determination, she assumed she could simply will herself to die, just as she had willed herself to live so long and so fully. So she took to her bed, never counting on the fact she had kept herself so healthy in body and mind that she couldn't just close her eyes and die. It took her a year to die, during which she could have enjoyed life. But she had no more pictures of a future. Someone once said depression is the absence of a future; I now make sure I am constructing a positive one constantly.

Before the time of her death, however, I met more of these phenomenal dancers. A teacher I had in New York, in her eighties at the time, came into class, still dressed for dancing. She would grasp the barre, step up onto the very tips of her toes, and unfold one leg at shoulder height. It seemed fairly remarkable at the time; now it seems astonishing. Another teacher in New York, a well-known male dancer, is still directing and making occasional appearances in walk-on roles, such as Herr Drosselmeyer in *The Nutcracker*. He was ninety-eight years old the last time I checked. These people seemed to be handing me a mandate—almost a trust that I must take care not to violate—to be healthy and long lived.

Then there was my great-grandfather, about whom I have heard so many stories. A tall, handsome man, he participated in many of the most well-known battles of the Civil War, and he was a member of the famous "Iron Brigade" that turned the tide at Gettysburg. He was wounded and left for dead three times during the war. Each time, he crawled off the battlefield and survived. My sister remembers when, as a little girl, she heard him tell his stories. About his near-death experiences, he turned to her and winked, saying, "I fooled 'em all." Great-Grandpa was jolly, good humored, and much loved by everyone around him. In his later years, he took to traveling around to visit relatives. Arriving unexpectedly, he would throw his hat in the door, saying, "If no one threw it out again, I knew it was all right to come on in."

I grew up as the youngest member of an aging family. Although my mother was only twenty-nine when I was born, my father was fifty-four. My father had no living immediate family members. We lived with my mother's parents. My mother's brother and sister were away in the armed forces during World War II, so the only relatives I saw on numerous family occasions were grandparents and great aunts and uncles. I was called "the little one" by a whole host of gray-haired people. I find that in any gathering, I still somehow think of myself as the youngest one there, although the fact that my seventy-fifth birthday is approaching makes that statement somewhat absurd! Still, it has always been my self-perception.

A major theme in my parents' philosophy was that we should hold to our self-perception and not be overwhelmed by someone else's authority or supposed knowledge. This included teachers, doctors, politicians, and so on. We were supposed to think for ourselves, rather than follow others people's leads. My mother had a favorite question, which she delivered in a challenging tone of voice, whenever we were about to fall victim to conformity: "Do you want to run with the herd?" We learned very early on that the only correct answer was, "No, of course not." So we always felt free to disagree (politely and sometimes privately) with our teachers and other authority figures. This stood us in good stead later on when we dealt with doctors, some of whom have delivered what might have been damaging blows to our self-perception.

For instance, I had a sore knee about forty years ago, and an orthopedic surgeon assured me I would need surgery. When I refused and instead demanded physical therapy, he signed the order reluctantly, saying, "You'll be back." Not only have I not gone back, but I can't even tell you now which knee it was. I dealt with the problem as I tend to do frequently, by taking charge and finding a more natural solution than what the "expert" recommended. It did require me to work (at the physical therapy exercises) rather than hand the problem over to an authority figure to fix.

In a similar vein, peer pressures haven't affected me at any stage in life. When I was young and people all around me were smoking, I refused to do so, thinking it was a dumb thing to do to your body. So many eating behaviors seemed to fall into that category, too. I wanted to be slim and fit, ready to meet any challenges life threw at me. Now that I'm older, I do not readily accept the discussions I hear from my age mates about the "inevitabilities" of aging. Upon reflection, I realize one reason peer pressure has not affected me is that I have never perceived my age mates as "peers." I had been taught to think—and act—for myself.

In my forties, I realized that I wanted to retire early and that it was important to plan not only for financial support but for continued support of friends and meaningful activities. I had seen older people retire, only to find they were very lonely. I determined that this would not happen to me. I immediately set about making new friends outside my circle at that time, focusing on people who would not be stuck in schedules preventing them from going out to "play" with me, whether for a day event or an international trip.

I also realized that I had a large appetite for life and that maybe I had better lay out in an organized way all the things I wanted to sample. For example, I had continued to dance even after becoming a college instructor, but by age forty-five, it was becoming painful and fatiguing. So I took up ballroom dancing, a less strenuous but still rewarding form of movement. I also knew I loved music and that my next step would be to study singing. To renew my studies of French language and culture, which I love, I went down to the Alliance Française the day after my early retirement. Then I combined my love of music and the French language to study French cabaret songs from the 1930s and 1940s.

I always knew I would get back to writing, which I had done as a child. It had always been a way to express my deepest thoughts in an organized way. I now write one e-zine article per week and am working on two books simultaneously—one on shyness and self-esteem, and the other on stress management for people who believe they are too busy to take care of themselves properly. At some point, I know I will take up drawing and painting, activities I loved as a child.

In looking at my list, I notice I have put the most vigorous activities first, gradually moving to those that take less energy and physical strength. But all of them involve life, and all of them involve learning and meeting new people. So it's really a plan to give up things I knew I would probably have to give up anyway, but to always replace them with something interesting, something to which I could look forward. I am reminded of a card someone once sent me with this quote from Molly Fumia: "Being alive requires of us a relationship with the mysterious life-long experience of letting go."

I was temporarily taken aback when, at age sixty-eight, I had a "heart attack that never should have happened." The sense of having violated that trust my dance "ancestors" had handed down to me was strong, and I felt ashamed. Moreover, I felt humiliated as a "stress solutions expert" (I had started a college class on the psychology of stress in the 1970s and had created the text for the course). It was a setback, one from which I took several years to recover psychologically. It profoundly affected my self-esteem.

I began to reflect carefully on what had brought me—someone who had always received praise from my doctors for my low blood pressure and excellent cholesterol numbers—to this place. I realized I had (rather arrogantly) assumed I had built up a huge health bank account, against which I could draw with impunity. So when I was hit with a cross-country move, plus the simultaneous caretaking of two failing older adults, not to mention some rather ugly legal episodes surrounding the death of one, I fell into what I call the "Stress Whirlpool," where disturbed sleep can exacerbate poor eating, feelings of fatigue and depression, and lack of exercise.

One of the other factors, besides what seemed to be overwhelming stress, was that I have an inherited factor in my blood, lipoprotein (a), that makes me three times more likely than the average person to have a heart attack. I believe I have some control over that factor—control I had relinquished because I wasn't paying attention.

But I have now taken charge of my life so well that my cardiologist believes I will not have another heart attack. Throughout this process of taking charge, I've started to think about the difference between "healing words" and "harmful words." For example, still bewildered after my heart attack, I asked the first cardiologist to whom I was assigned, "Why did this happen to *me*?" Her reply was, "It's just old age." I had never felt old, nor did I think I looked old. My self-image was that of a vibrant, attractive person deeply involved in life and acceptable everywhere I went. Suddenly, I felt gray and bent over, unattractive, and on a sure but possibly slow slide to death. I no longer seemed to have a future, and life seemed hopeless (a very damaging belief, as research now verifies).

It took me two years to get over the depression, even though my first move—a good one—was to fire that cardiologist and get a new one. The new one is excellent. It was she who ordered the test that revealed a large quantity of lipoprotein (a) in my blood. My personal research indicates that, at this time, there is no diet, medication, or exercise program that will lower the level of lipoprotein (a). When I asked my new cardiologist about lowering lipoprotein (a), her response was that of a fighter: "We don't have a solution for that—yet."

Her inclusion of that word *yet* is an important one. It suggests there is a future. It tells me she has faith that someone is working on the solution, and that because her mind is open to the possibility, she will learn about it as quickly as possible and just as quickly pass it on to me. This is the kind of person I want on my medical team, and I waste no time getting rid of anyone who doesn't exude healthy optimism.

By no means do I assume all my challenges will be solved by the medical profession. I do my part, every day. I scrutinize my diet, working hard to reduce the presence of "empty" foods (with little or no nutritional value), while increasing my intake of fruits and vegetables.

It hasn't been easy. The great quantities of chocolate I used to eat were far beyond the little amount that has been deemed "heart healthy." I thought I would feel badly deprived if I had to limit myself to one or two very small pieces per day. And ice cream—how could I do without a daily scoop of ice cream? Not the low-fat, ice milk, or frozen yogurt kind, but the real, full-cream stuff. I had also assumed for many years that the mere presence of a vegetable on my plate was sufficient.

Now I make sure at least half of my plate is covered with vegetables, and I have learned to cook them in more and more imaginative ways. One of the things I have found over time is that I actually crave vegetables, and the lure of chocolate and ice cream has decreased dramatically. My body has adjusted to good health.

And my response to that heart attack was that I was motivated to start a new business at age seventy-two, speaking and writing in the area of stress management and cardiac disease. I tell my story, "The Angina Monologue," over and over again to interested audiences, helping the overly busy, overly stressed people I see every day find what I call "islands of peace" in their daily lives; make better choices about what they eat, do, and think; and quickly shift their mindset from stressed to serene.

Once again, I feel vital and strong. My head is full of plans for the future, a future in which I travel and bring healthy and helpful messages to my audiences. My motto is this: I want to help people save their own lives, *and to make sure it's a life worth saving*.

I intend to savor my life for many more years, and inside of me, I feel an echo of my great-grandpa's phrase: "Ha, I fooled 'em all."

....

Conscientiousness...

Personality is the unique, relatively stable pattern of feelings, thoughts, and behavior each individual displays. There are five personality traits that describe human personality: openness, conscientiousness, extraversion, agreeableness, and neuroticism.

Lynette, like the participants in *The Longevity Project*, demonstrates a conscientious personality through her persistence and attention to detail. Research shows that people with this personality trait tend to take better care of themselves by actively staying on top of their health. Conscientious or not, however, if we allow others' needs to overshadow our own, we put our health at risk. This was the case for Lynette, and her choices resulted in the "heart attack that never should have happened."

Prioritizing is a key skill for conscientious living. When we prioritize correctly, our visions for life become reality. Lynette, for example, conscientiously includes in her schedule things that are important and of interest to her. She also purposefully gives order to her days and overall life. This is what makes Lynette and other conscientious people successful. They exhibit a degree of self-discipline by organizing their lives through daily routines.

Lynette had dreams and visions of a long, fulfilling life from a very young age. And she continues to keep dreaming, creating, and evolving. Whatever their dreams may be, thrivers cultivate communities that provide them with the support and encouragement they need to succeed. (Lynette, for example, replaced her initial cardiologist with one who better met her needs.)

Along with supporters, we may encounter nonbelievers and naysayers along the path to achieving our dreams. Sometimes these naysayers have innocent intentions, and sometimes not. Regardless, thrivers have learned not to allow these people to dash their enthusiasm, confidence, and vision. Thrivers stay strong and true to their dreams.

Lynette could have accepted her first doctor's answer when she asked, "Why did this happen to me?" But Lynette's ability to think for herself—a lesson she learned at a young age—helped her realize the doctor's reply ("It's just old age") was limited thinking. It was clear to Lynette that the statement did not align with her beliefs, values, or perception of herself; therefore, the statement was not true for her. Perspective is necessary when an unexpected event, such as Lynette's heart attack, derails your everyday life and thinking.

The perceived sense of control we feel over stressful events is a key factor in determining whether the event will create vulnerability or resilience. People who lack a sense of control often live by "if only" statements, which effectively prevent them from living in the present moment. The positive, healthy role models in Lynette's life seemed to strengthen her inner confidence to eventually write her own prescription for good health and vitality after her heart attack. Mentoring gives a person both roots and wings.

Lynette's conscientious approach to life teaches us that in order to thrive, we may need to challenge conventional thinking and push the boundaries of what's expected. Thrivers grow to become their own best advocates by stepping into their voices of power. Are you ready to be—at least occasionally—the nonconformist, the rule breaker, the one to shake things up to live your best life, just as Lynette has done?

Nadia Giordana
Age 64

Not long ago—at an age when in generations past I would have retired and spent my time lunching with friends, babysitting grandchildren, or perfecting my golf swing (all great things at the right place and time, especially grandchildren)—I decided to do something different with my life. That meant I needed to take a hard look at where I was; figure out how I had slipped off track; and determine what was missing, where I wanted to be, and how I was going to get there.

The first thing I did was work on my personal transformation. That meant losing weight—eighty-eight pounds, to be exact—which I did in a relatively short period of time, with healthy lifestyle changes and without fad dieting or surgery.

In the '70s as a young, twenty-something woman, I became a "health nut" at a time when it was considered offbeat to be eating whole foods and exercising. I embraced that lifestyle, and it worked for me. But even with this early imprinting on my health, the stresses of making my way through the tangled and competitive corporate world got the best of me, and in my mid-forties and into my fifties, the weight piled on. I carried it for a good, long time—about fifteen years. So when I decided to start losing it, it wasn't like losing nine months of baby weight. I was older, and my body was used to it and didn't want to change.

At age fifty-eight, I was laid off in a corporate downsize; it devastated me at the time, as I had planned to retire there. Perhaps being older and overweight hastened my demise? Whatever the reason for the layoff, I spent a year recovering, feeling useless, and wondering if I should just retire. Eventually, I decided I had a lot more living to do. That's when I set about losing the weight.

I didn't want to go on a structured diet; I knew that wouldn't work. My entire lifestyle and manner of thinking about food and life had to change. So I got back to my roots. I remembered what I had learned about healthy eating in years past, researched new information, studied several popular diets for the best of what they had to offer, and began a methodical changeover in my lifestyle. I replaced the bad habits I had acquired with good ones, one by one. I maintained a daily dialogue with God, and in that same mindset, I was keenly aware of the power of prayer, positive thinking, and visualization.

Using these basic tools every day, I reached my goal weight ten months later without the benefit of exercise. (I had a leg injury, partially due to being overweight, that initially prevented me from weight-bearing exercise.) But the momentum continued, and over the following four months, I added exercise to my routine and eventually reached my ideal weight—all this without ever going on a restricted diet. Today I maintain my healthy lifestyle and attitude, and my weight is no longer an issue.

During the months of the weight loss, I kept extensive notes and a food diary, thinking I might create a blog or write an article about my experiences. But as time went on, I realized I had the makings of a book. Not long after reaching my weight goals, I set about writing and publishing *Thinking Skinny: Transform Any Healthy Weight-Loss Program into Supercharged Success*. I eventually entered it in the 2009 Midwest Independent Book Awards, and it was a finalist in the May 2010 award ceremonies event.

As the second part of making a change in my life and doing something different, I decided to overcome a lifelong fear: I suffered from a deep-seated dread of public speaking. Inspired by my weight-loss success, I decided to climb that mountain, too. But working on my public-speaking ability was a bigger challenge than losing weight, and I didn't know where to start. (The truth is, this will be an ongoing endeavor.)

I started with one or two short speaking engagements and went from there with longer presentations. Then I began hosting an Internet radio show, where I interviewed extraordinary women. In addition to sharing my own wisdom, tips, and insights, I interviewed these women about their life-changing stories. I share some of them on my website, EmbodyYourVision.com. This helped me a lot, as the spotlight wasn't directly on me; I placed my focus on my guests. I was able to speak comfortably without becoming self-conscious. Later, I got interested in video and used it to film my personal website introductions and several of my subsequent presentations. Adding a video camera to the mix of tools helped me even more with my speaking skills.

Overcoming these two huge hurdles—losing weight and addressing my fear of speaking—made me feel younger, more alive, invincible, and unstoppable. How sad and full of regret would I have been had I lived my whole life and never conquered these things? I believe that whatever your age, it's never too late to shake off negative self-talk and reinvent new chapters in your life. One of my favorite quotes is from Edwin Louis Cole: "You don't drown by falling in the water; you drown by staying there."

Changing my life filled me with desire to help others change theirs. Some people would label me a coach, but that's not accurate. I'm more of a facilitator and mentor, a lifestyle strategist. My mission is to help women living the second act of their lives find the courage or inspiration they need to reawaken their deepest, most passionate dreams, and I help them define strategies to make those dreams happen. Because "someday" is here, and it's time for us to do the things we always said we were going to do.

I'm just like you. And like you, I've reinvented myself several times in my life—not always intentionally. It wasn't until someone pointed out to me that I had reinvented my life a number of times that I became consciously aware of what I was doing. From that moment, I began to reinvent with intent. I developed my own customizable **"Lifestyle GPS System"** that helps me write and create roadmaps for new adventures in my life. I have a saying: Lifestyle choices are a lot like buying new clothes. We try on different things until something fits, but even then, it doesn't fit forever, or it goes out of style, or we tire of it. It's up to us to discard a bad fit as soon as we recognize it.

As I consciously and intentionally reinvent myself, I realize the two people who have inspired me the most are my parents. That may sound like a gratuitous tipping of the hat, but not once you learn that in 1979, Norman and Sylvia Wilkins, at the age of fifty and after raising four children to adulthood, sold their dairy farm in Minnesota, loaded up a 1964 Freightliner semi-tractor and trailer with 73,000 pounds of gear and equipment, said goodbye to family and friends, and set out to carve a new life for themselves on the frozen tundra of Alaska.

They built a log cabin that early on had no electricity, water, or indoor plumbing. For twenty-seven years, they lived off the land and with what little income they had. Norman trapped, hunted, and prospected for gold, while Sylvia (all the time missing her children) made new friends and built a large garden in a forbidding and very short growing climate. Much of what she grew had to be started with the help of a greenhouse they built. She picked berries and made preserves; sewed and repaired clothing, sometimes by hand and with a treadle machine; cleaned and canned salmon; and dressed out, packaged, and prepared moose, bear, caribou, and other game.

All through those years, Norman chronicled their adventure in his daily journal entries. Recently, I transcribed those journals and published them as a three-volume docu-journal, *10,000 Days in Alaska*.

I never get tired of hearing them tell their stories,

and I've never lost my sense of amazement at what they have done. They are in their mid-eighties now and have reluctantly left Alaska to move back to Minnesota, due to health issues. Someday I would like to be as unique and full of adventure as they are. I expect that means I've got some surprises ahead of me. I wonder what they will be?

As I observed my parents' saga unfold, I began to awaken to the idea that one's later years can have tremendous potential. It instilled in me a longing for that sense of adventure and accomplishment that comes only from stretching oneself. If I'm different from other women at my age, I think it is my willingness to take risks and try things, knowing full well that I might end up looking foolish to some. I can live with that. I would say to you, in whatever decade you are living, find the magic in it.

I'm not even close to considering retirement or taking it easy. I would much rather be meeting and interacting with other talented women who are making their mark in this world, leaving a legacy, *doing* things.

My advice? Think of your best life as a book, and ask yourself, *what chapters are yet to be written?*

....

Adaptability, a Willingness to be Transformed...
Leaving something behind can be difficult, especially when we don't have a choice in the matter. But understanding that each step we take in our lives prepares us for the next can help turn a disappointment into a springboard for greater success. Thrivers are masters at reframing life's devastating blows. Nadia clearly demonstrates this. She turned a corporate layoff into a time for rediscovering her interest in health and fitness and a time for personal growth.

Transitions are not times when we lose our identities, but times when we can evolve a dimension of ourselves. A midlife transition, especially, can be enlightening or frightening; it all comes down to how we perceive or frame our situation. In general, midlife is simply a normal transition to another stage of life. Often, it's a time when people reevaluate their priorities, aspirations, and goals. Common focuses include recreation and pursuing dreams that may have been abandoned due to family or work-related obligations.

We can choose to view the stages of life as a "map" to the unknown territory through which we must move. Until recently, midlife transitions were completely "unmapped" and unacknowledged. But now, the timing of major life events has become less and less predictable at all levels of society. No one can really predict when exactly we will get married, have children, become grandparents or empty-nesters, enter the retirement stage, or launch ourselves back into a work or volunteer role. Giving up our rigid predictions for when life events or life transitions *should* occur is an important part of becoming a thriver. In fact, flexibility and adaptability are key traits of thrivers who achieve their AgePotential.

Nadia, for example, had intended to retire at the company from which she was eventually laid off. Like most people who incur a blow in life, Nadia was shaken to the core. She felt insecure and at times "useless." But she didn't linger in that state of mind—which is precisely what sets thrivers and non-thrivers apart. Instead of wishing for a different outcome, complaining, blaming, or harboring resentment, she chose to perceive her situation as a new challenge and opportunity for growth. Nadia didn't just go out and get another job; instead, she transformed herself and her life. Now, due to her experience with reinventing a new chapter in her life, she is currently mentoring other women to do the same.

Choosing to make a career change is one thing, and being forced to do so is another. A common business or life mantra is "Failing to plan is planning to fail," but planning to be flexible and adaptable may be the most life-enhancing wisdom anyone can give. Every exit is an entrance to somewhere else. When one door closes, another one opens. Nadia chose to relinquish what was, look forward to the new opportunity, and move on with her life.

Ultimately, she grew stronger in spite of the shocking blow. Are you prepared for your next life transition? Have you cultivated a strong sense of flexibility, just like Nadia?

Connie Goldman
Age 81

My name is Connie Goldman, and I've just celebrated my eighty-first birthday.

I wonder what your reaction was to my introduction, but I'll make a guess: Some of you may be thinking, "I'm only fifty-six, so I don't think someone that old can tell me what I need to know at this time of my life. I guess I'll just skip to the next chapter in this book." But no matter your age, your particular stage of life, or what you think you need to know about your upcoming life transitions, I may be able to offer you some insights and inspiration.

I'd like to begin by summing up the general attitude our culture has toward older adults with one word: *ageism*. Working in the area of human development for over thirty years, I have observed that the most prevalent attitude toward aging in this country is that you must do everything you can to stay young. Images of people in advertisements for clothing, vacation getaways, and even retirement communities look younger and younger. For whatever reason, Americans generally feel the best way to grow old is to strive to remain young, look ageless, and remain part of the busy and productive world out there.

Personally, I've had an extremely difficult time unlearning the "busy and productive" patterns of my earlier career days. I worked hard during that time to be valued, appreciated, and accepted. The pressure to excel required me, and others, to earn our value in society by "doing."

As I've aged, however, much of the "doing" that mattered to me then has been replaced by "being"—with self-exploration as a process of growing "whole." These days, silent walks in the woods and meditation have become experiences of greater value. I've also discovered gardening to be one of the best activities for self-reflection. I've worked with many individuals to explore what "grows" inside them when they dig, plant, and connect with the earth—and they've all found that gardening lends itself to "inner work." All of this has helped me embrace my current stage in life, but it has also led to a greater need to spend time alone. As silly as this may sound, it has led me to want to "share myself with me."

Ageism made it difficult for me to learn how to value simply "being." But what if we all embraced our age and stage in life, no matter our circumstances?

How different would the future look if you concerned yourself less with what you might lose and concerned yourself more with what you might gain? How would we live our later years if we didn't focus only on growing old but if we explored ways to grow whole? What if we perceived aging not as a disease to be cured but as a normal life process that may even offer rewards?

Perhaps it was more natural for me, after all, than it will be for others to adjust to this way of thinking about aging. Through my work as a writer, speaker, and public radio producer and reporter, I've devoted myself to projects and programs exclusively concerned with the challenges and changes we experience in midlife and beyond. And in doing so, I have been fortunate to meet many older adults who helped me discover a new way to view the process of aging—one in stark contrast to the American idea of aging. My life would not be the same without the influence of these role models.

Even so, I believe the challenge for each of us is to figure out how we can age in a more life-affirming, accepting, and satisfying manner. I believe it's possible to view the aging process as an opportunity to continue learning, to expand our vision, to find great satisfaction in new activities, to gain a deeper understanding of ourselves, and to explore who we are today. We all need to deal with changes, challenges, and transitions at certain points throughout our lives. I believe each of those hurdles offers an opportunity for us to understand ourselves better.

Let me share a life experience that was told to me in an interview with the late educator and columnist Eda LeShan. I believe her words offer a profound insight into a philosophy of embracing our individual aging process, dealing with it, growing with the years.

It was a time in my life when I was thinking about writing a book about middle age. I was at a social event, and I was introduced to an oceanographer who started a conversation with me, asking if I knew that lobsters have to de-shell. He told me that they get crowded inside their three-pound shells and they're uncomfortable, and it's not possible for them to go on living if they stay in the shells. So what they do is go out to the seas unprotected. The might get eaten by another lobster or a large fish, but they must de-shell. The whole, hard shell comes off, and the pink membrane that's inside grows and eventually becomes a harder shell and a bigger one.

At first, that story didn't hit me, but soon I became preoccupied thinking about lobsters. I even was dreaming about them. One day I told my ther-

apist about my lobster dreams. And she replied, "That's exactly what you're writing your book on middle age about…going to the reef and taking off your familiar shell even if it's dangerous." That has become my philosophy of life. You know, if you stay stifled where you are, you're dead before you're dead.

I've learned that the thing you need most as you age is the courage of a lobster. You're going to go through things where you have to become much more flexible. You have to be willing to change, and courage is the most essential part of it. I believe courage implies a lack of denial, that you really are willing to face the issues, whatever they are, and that you grow from them. There's nothing that happens to you as long as you're alive that you don't learn from. And that has been my philosophy of life, at any age, and it certainly is now. You know, if you stay stifled where you are, you're dead before you're dead.

LeShan contended that our transition years are full of uncertainty, but we must make necessary changes and let go, even if we're frightened or uncertain. Losing your job, children growing up and leaving home, having an unexpected responsibility of caring for an ill or aging family member, dealing with your own health changes, or any circumstance in one's life requires change, adjustment, or letting go of the familiar. There's meaning and familiarity in the regularity of our lives and in our self-image related to our work; our role in our community, church, and synagogue; or the various roles others have come to recognize as our identity. I've personally learned to let go of some of the "doing" part of my life and reflect upon who I am now; I'm no longer who I was.

I believe what Eda meant is that as you age, you can grow and learn when you make even small changes, larger ones, and even leaps. So many hang on to an attitude that remaining active, distracted, and constantly busy is superior to taking the time for reflection, introspection, or contemplation. Yet it takes getting to know and understand a different relationship to the self, and that often requires quiet time with oneself.

Yes, I too often avoid change—just like everyone else—and sometimes my avoidance doesn't make a difference in any given situation. But there have been times in my life when my instinct, or my "gut," has told me to make a change. Sometimes I'm afraid to say yes to what seems like a big change, but when I'm down to the wire and I realize holding back isn't a wise or practical choice, I let go of the old and move on. Several times in my life I've come to a place where I'm able to say to myself, "Okay, I'll move on," and with some apprehension and often actual fear I push through the resistance. Decisions, changes, and complex transitions need some serious thinking like a lobster, to shed the old shell and move on. In fact, I too have learned that the thing a person needs most as they age is the courage of a lobster.

I know from my own experience that we inevitably go through situations that require us to become much more flexible, and courage will be essential. I've often worked hard to summon the courage to willingly face the issues, whether big or small, and open the opportunity to grow in new ways as I embrace the necessary changes.

I believe nothing happens to us that we can't learn from. Throughout my career, I've worked with many persons in midlife and older adults, and they've told me how they grew to know themselves better in late life. Most described becoming wiser and more focused. I've personally learned too that there are opportunities to learn from every life transition. Some of my life events, and most probably yours, have been stressful, anxiety provoking, and difficult. Others are satisfying, rewarding, and joyous. Yet I find with aging that I've experienced new learning and growing and knowing myself in new ways. My philosophy at every age, but more than ever now, is as Eda LeShan told me: if you stay stuck, you're dead before you're dead.

....

Embrace the Aging Journey...

To despair growing older actually makes you grow old faster, while to accept growing older with grace may actually help you avoid the physical and mental health problems often associated with the aging process. Connie challenges us to consider the journey of growing older as something of value—as a time to grow "whole." To grow whole implies that an individual has more to discover, more evolution to undergo, and more *life* to *live*.

Each stage in life has a distinct purpose. The second half of life may be a time to integrate our life experiences or create (or recreate) something new. It may be a time to ask ourselves what we have left undone or undeveloped within ourselves. It's a time to ask, "What does being whole mean to me?" This requires reflection and involves a conscious effort to stop "doing" and instead find inner stillness by "being," at least occasionally. But "being" and "doing" are equally important for our self-development and journey to becoming whole. Without one or the other, we would live superficially.

Connie, like most thrivers, understands the importance of striking a balance between "doing" and "being." For example, the title of one of her books, *Who Am I...Now That I'm Not Who I Was?*, explains how our identity, purpose, and priorities will shift over time. Wholeness, in fact, is a journey of self-exploration. Connie learned this, in part, through her professional work, which mainly focused on midlife and beyond. By reflecting on the thrivers' life stories contained within my book, you can do the same.

When it comes to growing older, Connie also teaches us to embrace it—not to "succumb" to it. After all, our youthfulness does not lie in our chronological age but instead somewhere between "being" and "doing." Contrary to what people think, growing whole means putting our energy and mindfulness into living abundantly at every age.

The first confrontation with age comes with separation from the familiar. We must welcome the unexpected changes in life. Resistance is futile, but it is a deeply ingrained habit. Instead, learn to bend with grace and humility. Grow through it all, and never ever forget to notice the beauty change can bring. If you consider each stage in life as an opportunity for growth, rather than something to be resisted, avoided, or dreaded, then you will live from a place of wholeness.

How will you harness the courage of a lobster, as Connie states, to balance "doing" and "being" in your life—and, ultimately, to live out your AgePotential?

Fran Heitzman, as told to Mary Fran Heitzman
Age 86

Early one morning, in the midst of the Great Depression of the 1930s, my aunt France sat on her front steps. With her back hunched and elbows pressed into her thighs, she bowed her head and covered her face with her hands. *Dear God,* she wondered, *what will I feed my family today—the cupboard and the icebox are bare!* After several minutes of complete despair, Aunt France looked up. A slight breeze ruffled something in the road. The "something" was a rabbit no longer alive, but still holding the warmth of life. Out of complete desperation, Aunt France fixed rabbit stew for supper.

In every generation there are "haves" and "have-nots." Aunt France was a "have-not." My family and my friends were "have-nots." The "haves" slept in clean, warm beds and had plenty of food on the table. The rest of us lived a more day-to-day existence. But you know, I seldom felt dejected as a kid because everyone in my immediate circle was no better off than us. We simply didn't know any better, as we didn't know real prosperity. We were happy, ordinary kids.

But I do remember one Christmas Eve that looked awfully bleak. We didn't expect a thing—nothing—because we knew there were no more ways to stretch what little we had. My dad shoveled coal for a dollar a day, and my mom, as many mothers did, cut adult clothes down to size and restitched them to fit us kids. That year, ours would be a Christmas without a tree or presents.

I was just seven years old, and I'll never forget the knock on the door all those years ago. My mom pulled the window curtain aside to see who might be at our house on Christmas Eve. We weren't expecting anyone. And there stood Grandma Bradbury, wrapped in layers against the cold. Now, Grandma Bradbury was not my grandmother and not related to our family in any way. She lived down the road and worked for Hennepin County of Minnesota. Her garage was full to the rafters with food, clothing, and household items all of us "have-nots" relied on.

And on that Christmas Eve, Grandma Bradbury had a Christmas tree in one hand and a bag of oranges in the other. You can't even imagine how excited we kids were to see that Christmas tree *and* oranges. In those days, we rarely ever had fresh fruit in the wintertime, other than the apples we had picked in the fall and kept in the cellar.

Grandma Bradbury had a heart for what she did. Putting smiles on children's faces and relaxing the creases of stress on their parents' faces was as much a part of her job as keeping track of bureaucratic paperwork. Trudging through snow banks on a bitterly cold Christmas Eve was as thrilling for her as it was for us to receive her kindness and bounty.

That Christmas tree and those oranges laid the groundwork for the project I launched when I was sixty-one years old. You see, my wife, Jeanne, and I had raised seven kids. We never lived in luxury, but we always had food on the table and a roof over our heads. I'd owned and operated a drycleaners and later a landscaping business. Eventually, I retired from entrepreneurship and worked as the chief maintenance man at our church, Pax Christi, in Eden Prairie, Minnesota. Our lives were comfortable. *We* had become the "haves."

In those early days of my work at church, a parishioner stopped by one afternoon and asked, "Do you know of anyone who is in need of a baby crib? I've got one to give away."

"We'll take it!" I said, and I headed off to her car and lugged that thing in. After the kind lady left our church parking lot, I got right to work and called Catholic Charities. "Do you need a baby crib, I asked?" Their response echoed mine: "We'll take it!"

And then my long-ago memories of Aunt France's desperation and Grandma Bradbury's tireless dedication resurfaced. *Why can't we, today's "haves," bridge the gap between us and the "have-nots"?*

And that was the beginning of Bridging, Inc., a nonprofit I founded that takes the desperation out of people's lives. In addition to all manner of household goods, we supply beds, mattresses, and warm blankets for those in transition. The recipients might be new to our country; temporarily out of work; rebounding from a house fire, natural disaster, or illness; or maybe they've simply fallen through society's cracks. Whatever their circumstances, we are the bridge that offers hope and a second chance.

But while my passion for Bridging burned, my own life was nearly snuffed out by a major health crisis. I've never used drugs or had any addictions, but I could have taken better care of myself. My morning bacon and daily doughnut habit contributed to some very clogged arteries! At age sixty-seven, persistent clutching pains in my chest resulted in a 4:00 a.m. phone call to my son. Soon we were speeding through red lights and dodging early-morning traffic. Not long after we arrived at the hospital, I was wheeled into an operating room for quintuple bypass surgery.

Before the sedation took hold, I had a quick talk with the Almighty: "Dear God," I said, "if you'll give me just a little more time, I'll work real hard for you." Well, the Lord must have figured I'd be good on my promise. I came through that surgery and recovered on schedule. I returned to my job at church and to my passion, Bridging, with renewed energy and enthusiasm.

Today, Bridging serves 115 households a week, via a small paid staff and over 6,000 individual and group volunteers who give 84,000 hours of their time annually. Most recipients who come to the Bridging warehouse are referred by one of over 130 social service agencies. One of the first things we make sure each person receives is a solid bed to sleep in and plenty of blankets to keep warm. Assuring a good night's sleep is just one of many ways we renew people's hope.

At eighty-six years of age, I'm grateful for the extra time I've been given. The smiles on kids' faces and the relief in their parents' eyes gives purpose to my life and energy to my days. Advancing age is not an excuse. Neither is it a death sentence. It's an opportunity—an opportunity to develop a zest for life that puts purpose into each day by touching the lives of others. When you wake up in the morning, thank God for the day ahead. Then figure out what your passion is, and give it all you've got.

....

Gratitude...

Thrivers are full of gratitude. The kindness bestowed upon Fran and his family, through gifts such as the Christmas tree and bag of oranges, made a profound, lifelong impact. It is evident that he carried a heart-felt sense of gratitude through the course of his life, no matter whether he was a "have" or "have-not."

Fran and others like him are a testament to the fact that people who thrive later in life do not neces-sarily come from a legacy of comfort, ease, or wealth. No matter our financial status, devoting ourselves to service helps us thrive and evokes feelings of gratitude, because it helps us realize how fortunate we are.

The phrase "It's more rewarding to give than to receive" may be a mere cliché to some, but not to Fran. If you've met him, you know he has never sought recogni-tion or an accolade. No, the impact he has had on others is his reward and source of happiness. In fact, research shows a clear connection between long-term happi-ness and gratitude, especially within families of mod-est means. What's more, a giving spirit such as Fran's spreads virally, touching the lives of people he may never meet, in ways he may never have imagined. That is the power of giving and the ticket to changing the world.

Just like Fran, grateful people tend to live lives devoted to "giving back." To my mind, Fran embodies the concept of *Pay It Forward*. *Pay It Forward,* a novel by Catherine Ryan Hyde that has also been made into a movie, illustrates how giving can spread virally. The main character, Trevor, has a plan to create a charitable program based on networking good deeds. He calls his plan "Pay It Forward," which means the recipient of a favor does a favor for a third party rather than paying the original favor-giver back.

We have all felt grateful and inspired in our lives, whether the inspiration came from our own experiences or others'. Feeling inspired is a basic human emotion—and helps us feel alive. We all know what to do when we feel inspired: give it away! Inspiration is not ours to keep. In fact, there is no benefit in holding onto it. So are you ready to be an inspiration, just like Fran, and pay it forward?

Jerry Johncock
Age 84

When I was fifty years old, my three youngest sons asked me to join them in running an eight-mile road race—but the race was only one month away. I knew I would need at least a few months to train for that distance, so I told them I'd run through the next spring and be ready for a race by late summer. Come August, I was geared up to hit the pavement, and I did—I finished third in the over-fifty age group!

I was thrilled to discover what would become a lifelong passion. I ran more and more, and gradually I was able to increase my speed and distance. By age sixty-one, my marathon time dropped under three hours and one minute—twice.

Running for fun quickly became a very healthy habit. Along with better physical fitness came other health benefits: I lost twenty pounds, and over time, my blood pressure dropped from 140/90 to 120/60, what's considered a normal reading for most adults. I was inspired to eat better, so I cut down on fats and refined food and upped my intake of vitamins and minerals. I'm now a firm believer that everyone should pay attention to their nutrition and do some form of vigorous exercise at least three or four days every week. The value of running is high at any age, and as they say, "If you don't use it, you'll lose it."

Maintaining a healthy lifestyle really hasn't ever been a challenge for me. When I was young, my father had a difficult relationship with alcohol, which persisted for many years and nearly ruined our family. But Mom prayed for Dad, and he eventually gave up alcohol—and cigarettes, too. He taught us to work hard, to be honest, and to have the confidence to succeed. The changes I observed in him were so good that I chose never to drink or smoke, and I'm glad to have made responsible choices for my health. If we misuse our bodies, we age rapidly. I've witnessed a handful of childhood friends destroy their lives with alcohol and die at a young age. It's such a shame.

During those early years, I knew Jesus answered Mom's prayers by helping Dad overcome his addictions. Watching her, I began to understand the value of faith. Mom was my mentor, my source of faith, love, and encouragement. She taught me to cast all my cares onto Jesus, to look to Him for support.

Today, my faith in Jesus helps me cope with life in many ways and has even influenced my running.

About nine years ago, I saw a T-shirt that said, "Run with Jesus." I liked it so much that I paid to have it printed in large red letters on both the front and back of my running shirt. It was the best five bucks I've ever spent. I wore that shirt in the 2008 Twin Cities Marathon. A race official mentioned to me that the overall record holder wore a shirt bearing the same message a few years before, and Jesus blessed me in a similar way that day: I broke the marathon national record of 4:13:00 with a time of 3:59:12 for the eighty-to-eighty-four age group.

I had some other big successes that year, such as breaking the thirty-kilometer national record by four and a half minutes in Milford, Michigan. And then on December 31, 2010, I broke the fifty-kilometer national record in Morganton, North Carolina, by sixty-four minutes with a 5:55 time.

My marathon and fifty-kilometer records were ratified December 2011 by USATF. It's much easier to break records at age eighty than at forty or fifty, because the competition drops off fast. But for me, the competition is still motivating; it gives me a vision for the future. I often look forward to moving into the next age group (for eighty-five to eighty-nine-year-olds) in 2013, so I will be among the "younger" runners in that group.

I still enjoy setting challenges for myself. For

instance, I've run 114 marathons and hope to compete in 200 by the end of my running career. It is also incredibly fulfilling when I help someone who feels like quitting before the finish—I've gained some lasting friendships through those encouraging interactions.

When it's me who feels discouraged, though—while running races or at other times—I turn to Jesus as well as my wife of fifty-eight years, my five sons, and my seventeen grandchildren. I know Jesus gives me constant peace of mind, and I know my loving family is always ready to help, under any circumstance. I look to our youngest son, Mark, who often drives me to my races, for encouragement and support on race days. Another son, Bill, who is also a runner and a podiatrist, serves as my running coach and trainer. The Lord has blessed me with good health, and my running injuries have been slight. But when injuries happen, Bill provides guidance on how to care for them and usually has me up and running in less than three weeks! Needless to say, running has become a family affair, and for the past thirty-plus years, my wife and sons have given me tremendous support while I've pursued my passion.

At midlife, I didn't think eighty was "old" because my great-grandmother died at age 104. I'm now past eighty, but I feel different from my peers because I have a passion for running, a loving family, a supportive church, and, most importantly, faith in Jesus. I can confidently say my greatest strength is having Jesus and His spirit in my life. The Lord has given me good health, and I plan to keep on until I reach one hundred years or more. If I ever have to stop running, I'll find some other form of exercise. But until then, whenever I'm not running, I'll be planning my next run! My life's journey has taught me that if you use what you have and keep up your faith in Jesus, you'll never be sorry.

....

Spirituality

The goal of living a long life is not just to add more candles to a birthday cake. Instead, it is to continue seeking purpose and meaning, no matter our circumstances. Aging is not a curse; it is a natural process of life. And for those who have a strong sense of faith, aging is ultimately a spiritual journey. People who lead spiritual lives are often happier than those who may not have developed their spirituality.

The ability to thrive entails a holistic approach to life—where the mind, body, *and* spirit are all cared for. You can see how Jerry's life emulates that idea. Holistic health is based on the idea that the body, mind, and spirit are interdependent. This belief suggests that an imbalance in any one of these facets can affect the remaining two.

Earlier in the book, I discussed how the mind directly affects the body, and research also indicates that the body can, in turn, affect the mind. When the body gets physically fitter, so does the mind. According to John Ratey of Harvard Medical School, "I call exercise 'Miracle-Gro for the brain.' Exercise keeps brain cells healthy in a way that playing chess and other highly cognitive activities do not."

Although it is often ignored, our spiritual health is vital to our overall health and vitality. In other words, neglecting the spirit may contribute to physical and/or emotional disease, while caring for the spirit can result in physical and/or emotional well-being. According to Peter J. Weiss, MD, author of *More Health, Less Care*, "When you are spiritually healthy, you understand that *you matter* and are part of something much larger than yourself."

The meaning of life is to give life meaning. Jerry finds meaning in and through his relationship with Jesus. Jerry and most thrivers who have a deep sense of spirituality are strengthened by the knowledge that they are not alone in this journey called life. Jerry literally wears this sentiment on his sleeves, with his "Run with Jesus" T-shirt. You might compare the belief in a loving, supportive, and forgiving higher power to a positive mental coping mechanism. It's like having someone to turn to during discouraging times—somewhere to lay down the burdens of life.

Jerry's passion for running and his strong spiritual life appear to keep him living in an optimal, holistic state of being: happy, healthy, and passionate. Like Jerry, won't you begin to create a balanced life honoring your mind, body, and spirit to master the art of thriving?

Marjorie Johnson
Age "39"

In my mind, I never think about my chronological age. I only think about how I feel, and that is forever young. It all began the day I heard Jack Benny declare he was thirty-nine on a television program, only to have his wife interject he was thirty-nine last year, too. I thought, "What a clever idea. When I get to be thirty-nine, I am going to do the same." So started my philosophy of life and why I always feel young. In my mind, I will always be thirty-nine. Therefore, since I *think* I am only thirty-nine, there is nothing I cannot do. There is a saying, "Life begins at forty." Well, then, I haven't even begun to live!

When I really did turn thirty-nine, I was married to my wonderful husband, Lee, and we had two daughters and one son. I was in good health, enjoying life, and at a healthy weight. I liked my life at thirty-nine and was pleased with my lifestyle and who I was. I wanted nothing to change, and it hasn't. I depend upon myself to make that happen.

To maintain the mind and body of a thirty-nine-year-old, I decided to keep myself in the same shape I was then. I continue to exercise, eat healthy, get my eight hours of needed sleep, and keep a vital interest in everything and everybody. This chosen frame of mind has resulted in the energy, enthusiasm, and zest for life I had at thirty-nine. All my good habits have kept me in wonderful health, with none of the aches and pains other older people have.

I have come to realize how powerful the mind is. My mind and the way I choose to think and perceive my world dictates my life, not any age number. Most people focus on their chronological age, and that is such a mistake—so depressing. No wonder why people dread adding years to their life. In calendar years, I am growing older, but not in my mind. It doesn't matter if you look older, as long as your mind stays young.

Throughout my life, I've learned to embrace the opportunities around me. When we were newly married, Lee and I spent three years in occupied Japan, while Lee served as a dentist in the army and later the air force. It was a wonderful experience as I immersed myself in the art of oil painting, water coloring, and dress and pattern making. The student in me loved to learn and I found myself drawn to study the Japanese language, public speaking, and art history.

Over the years, I also learned that the younger

you are, the better it is to start saving and planning for what you want your future to be. It takes effort to reach your potential and goals. You are responsible for your life. If you want to achieve your goals, it requires a commitment to a life of work, time, and sacrifice. Life does not owe you anything. I learned that lesson at ten years old. I babysat, and I decided to save my money for something I wanted in the future, rather than spend it immediately for instant gratification. And that outlook has paid off. Later, Lee and I both worked our way through college at the University of Minnesota. Thanks to those years of hard work and going without many things, we now have a life that includes everything we desire. Every year since continues to be the *best*. What a wonderful thing life is!

My mother's advice, to do my very best at whatever I did, has become the foundation of how I live my life. When other people were retiring at age sixty-five, I was just starting my career, sharing my love of baking and life as I became a frequent guest on various local and national TV talk shows. It all began when the children were in high school, and I finally had time to enter my baking into the Minnesota State Fair to see if it was worthy of winning the highest honor, the Blue Ribbon. I entered four baking items and was thrilled to receive three ribbons. I was hooked. Wanting to produce winning entries, I kept increasing the number of items I entered, and the ribbons kept mounting. I continued to win Blue Ribbons at every fair thereafter and soon was asked to be on local television to demonstrate my ribbon-winning recipes. I published my winning recipes in my cookbook, *The Road to Blue Ribbon Baking with Marjorie,* so everyone can learn from all my secrets and be a blue ribbon baker, too.

Not only did the ribbons keep accumulating, but so did my television appearances. In 1996, I was invited to represent Minnesota in the James Beard Foundation's "Fairs Across the Country" event in New York. The event chairman took me up on my offer to help promote the event on television. While on a local New York TV station promoting this event, the producer for *The Rosie O'Donnell Show* saw me and invited me to be on the show. Rosie and her viewers liked me so much, I continued to be a guest until she ended her show in 2002. This was about the time *The Wayne Brady Show* began to air, and I was a guest a total of twenty-five times during the show's two-year run.

In 2006, Rosie was cohost of *The View,* and she asked me to be on that show. On my first appearance on *The View,* I drew the attention of yet another producer and was asked to be on *The Tonight Show.* I've been on the show sixteen times to date. In February

2011, I was a guest on *The Dr. Oz Show*. Being such a fan of Dr. Oz, I was thrilled to be asked back again in August. The most recent invitation was to be on the *The Rosie Show* on Oprah's network, OWN.

I find that being a talk-show guest is a fun, exciting experience. I take these opportunities seriously and work hard to be my best on the shows. I love to speak, and I never run out of things I want to tell the audience. The feedback from all my television and speaking appearances are so complimentary, it makes me feel great.

I am too busy having a wonderful life to give up a moment to think about my age. I just feel ageless. I wake up each day feeling wonderful, eagerly anticipating what new and interesting things are in store for me. You can, too!

I still have my wonderful husband, who is now retired, and three successful children. (Our oldest daughter is an aerospace engineer, and our second daughter and son are both physicians.) I am enjoying such good health and having such a fabulous, interesting life that I want to live forever. I realize that is not possible, but I am still working on it!

....

Healthy Perception of Self...

Psychological age can be defined as "where the age you feel meets the age you are." Do you think of yourself as young? True, your chronological age matters, but it's your interpretation of your age that has far-reaching implications for the aging process.

According to a study in *Journal of Gerontology: Psychological Sciences*, older adults tend to feel about thirteen years younger than their chronological age. Marjorie, however, states, "In my mind, I will always be thirty-nine." Marjorie discovered early on that the fountain of youth lies within herself—within her thoughts and belief system. Marjorie may or may not be aware of the new science called epigenetics, but she is well aware of her mind-body connection and how her self-perceptions contribute to her ability to remain active, healthy, and engaged in a meaningful and purposeful way well into late life. Understanding the power of the mind-body connection is essential for living out AgePotential, a concept that is missing from conversations about aging today. How we think and perceive our environment profoundly affects our health and lifelong well-being. Indeed, the mind's well-being holds the key to overall well-being.

In other words, being "youthful" is twofold: mental and physical. Most people are aware of the importance of maintaining a healthy body through diet and exercise in order to stay physically young; however, most people are less aware of the equal importance of maintaining mental youthfulness by viewing age as a number, not as an excuse or limitation. Feeling young psychologically is directly related to living an authentic, passionate life. Marjorie is clearly passionate about life and has taken the responsibility for creating the kind of life that allows her to say, "I wake up each day feeling wonderful, eagerly anticipating what new and interesting things are in store for me."

Your youthful state—in both body and mind—isn't in jeopardy just in old age, but at any age or time when you let go of those things that keep you biologically youthful. This includes, for instance, exercise, a plant-based diet, managed stress, new learning opportunities, new experiences, optimism, curiosity, and a zest for life. As our society moves increasingly toward a sedentary lifestyle—with less creative play; more fast-food; and more incidents of depression, stress, anxiety, obesity, and diabetes in young people—we have a new generation of people who are young chronologically, but old biologically and psychologically.

But Marjorie's youthful disposition has kept her

young, despite her chronological age. Positive emotions and perceptions such as this are not trivial; they are critical for living your best life. Like Marjorie, how will you change your self-perception to help you stay healthy and feeling young well into late life?

Jeff Noel
Age 53

No man on my dad's side of the family has lived past sixty. This fact, as you might imagine, has instilled me with a sense of urgency to live each moment to the fullest. So, from a young age, I've done my best to do just that, to make every moment count.

At age eighteen, for instance, I started a habit of living consciously and thinking in advance about the possible outcomes of my choices. I've made about a million choices since then, but a few big ones have shaped who I've become today. I left my family behind in Gettysburg, Pennsylvania, and went west for college. As a freshman at the University of Idaho, I decided to read everything I could about success and positive thinking, and I enrolled in the Disney World College Program.

Soon after college, I rode my bicycle across the country, and when I returned, I sought employment at a great company. I landed a job at Disney World. On my way to and from work and at home before bed, I listened to motivational tapes of visionary speakers such as Brian Tracy, Zig Ziglar, and Napoleon Hill every day. During those years, I decided I'd wait to marry the right person, and sure enough, with a little patience, I found her.

Still at Disney World, I married my wife, Cheryl, and we bought our dream lot behind the Magic Kingdom in 1990. Two years later, when I was thirty-three, we built the home we continue to live in today, and we began making efforts to have a child. Little did we know at the time, however, that our desire to become parents would lead us to face one of the most significant challenges of our lives.

From the time I was thirty-three to the time I was forty-one, we spent our life savings on in vitro fertilization (IVF), even though the process couldn't guarantee a child. When we were unsuccessful on our fifth IVF cycle and the odds of having a child looked bleak at best, I had the epiphany of a lifetime: I suddenly realized material things don't matter at all. Between our first and fifth IVF attempt, I had endured the kind of pain and emptiness that will bring you to your knees. Even though the prospect of being a dad scared the heck out of me at first, by our fifth try, I knew I was born to be a dad—but I also knew my chance at fatherhood was slipping away. Then, miraculously, we conceived our son on the sixth attempt. In the end, IVF not only gave us a son, but it also gave me a better understanding of what faith, hope, and love really mean.

After that sixth IVF cycle, life kept improving. At age forty, I was invited to become a speaker on leadership and professional development at central Florida's largest employer. Now, thirteen years later, I've spoken to nearly a million people from every walk of life and professional background imaginable. It has been a tremendous experience. I'm committed to "walking the talk"—that is, to embodying the ideas I present as a speaker—and the blessing I've discovered is that to teach is to learn twice.

But we all encounter setbacks from time to time. Adversity doesn't develop character; it reveals it. It would be unfair to not tell you two important, life-altering experiences that occurred in between some really great moments in life. The first was a painful self-discovery, prompted by a burning desire to be an example and not a warning. The painful revelation was that I either drink alcohol every day, or not at all—there is no middle ground. The second was discovering that our son, then five, has an incurable disease. Life goes on and is never easy, but it is glorious and worth the effort.

In another example of facing adversity, I had a major health scare after the promotion. My doctor discovered dangerous cholesterol levels, and he instructed me to exercise and change my diet. The warning prompted me to run the distance between two mailboxes every day for one week, then run the distance between three mailboxes every day during the second week, and so on. In my neighborhood, mailboxes are one hundred meters apart. So after one month, my run was equivalent to one lap around a high school track, but my pace was slower than walking—for real.

I continued exercising regularly, but every three years or so, boredom, apathy, self-pity, and a variety of other excuses crept into my thoughts about exercise and eating. I kept on, however, using the creative tactics to stay motivated that I teach in the classroom at Sunday school and at Disney. Eventually my pace quickened, my cholesterol levels normalized, and in 2009, I went on to represent the USA at the Masters Track and Field World Championships in the 400 meters!

How did I do it? I dared to ask myself these questions: *Why can't I? Why don't I try?* I believe you should never set limits for your health. It's better to be an example of good health at the end of your life than to be an example of bad health; in other words, we should all strive to model good health for the young people in our lives.

With my health back on track, I continued my quest to live each moment to the fullest, and I founded Mid

Life Celebration, LLC, at age forty-nine. The company challenges male baby boomers to do something great before they die, whether that means mending an important relationship, funding research for the treatment of a disease, or doing anything in between. At Mid Life Celebration, LLC, my dream is to teach personal responsibility in five key areas: mind, body, spirit, money, and HQ (the paperwork of life). I'm two years away from retiring from Disney, and when I give notice, I will put 110 percent of my effort toward Mid Life Celebration. In the meantime, I write five blogs every day—one in every key area—to get my message out.

While the six thousand blog posts I've published may set me apart from my peers in one way, my predisposition for envisioning my future and then making it happen is really what makes all the difference. I don't just hope things will happen; I make them happen. I am, after all, the "CEO of Jeff."

That said, I don't think I'm all that different from the rest of society. I've always believed it isn't death itself that we fear, but rather we fear not *living* before we die. Most people are afraid to fail and are therefore afraid to try. Many become self-conscious because they look to external influences to define their way of life, and as a result, they conform to society and fail to achieve their full potential. Fear of success is also a real phobia. The thought of what we are capable of can be scary. It is for me.

But that's what inspires me to think of *carpe diem* as a daily, moment-to-moment battle cry. The best path toward success and the best way to nurture self-growth, I've found, is to develop a sense of obligation to humanity. I truly believe everyone needs to find purpose in life, for without purpose, you will drift and flounder.

At fifty-three years old, I'm proud to say I feel a strong sense of purpose. My wife and I have been married for twenty-nine years, and our son is now eleven years old. I would love to be a grandfather someday, so I plan to take care of my mind and body in order to do so. Currently, I'm living out a ten-year plan that will take me to age sixty, and at that time, I will reassess my goals and strategies. Life can change on a dime, so one needs to be flexible. My greatest desire is for my life to demonstrate how to live and age well and to hear the following words during my last breath: "Well done, good and faithful servant."

....

Compelling Future...
Midlife, for most of us, is the first time we seriously consider our own mortality. Due to the legacy of his

father's family, Jeff considered his mortality at a young age. But instead of succumbing to the belief that he would die before age sixty—just as every other male on his father's side had done—he chose to use his family's health history as a warning and as motivation to proactively make the most of every moment. Jeff and thrivers alike may not get to choose everything that happens to them in life; however, they do have the ability to choose how they will respond.

According to Daniel G. Amen, MD, author of *Magnificent Mind at Any Age*, "Your brain is the most powerful organ in the universe. It has the ability to direct your life in a positive way or create a living hell. To harness your brain's power it needs direction and vision. It needs a blueprint." Vision is power. People who achieve their AgePotential always have a plan and a vision for the future.

Jeff clearly has both a plan and a vision for a fulfilling future: he's already laying the groundwork for his next dream project called Mid Life Celebration, even before he completes his time at Disney. Instead of fretting over his upcoming life transition, Jeff eagerly maps out the next. As the "CEO" of his life, Jeff intentionally plans his next step with purpose and meaning.

AgePotential requires a vision for a desirable future. In order to thrive, you *must* align your life with a deep understanding of purpose, mission, and vision. Only then will you continue to grow and evolve. You may wonder what happens when growth ceases. Stagnation and decay set in immediately. In other words, if you are not growing and expanding, you are basically beginning to die.

A sense of purpose to achieve the future you envision serves as the bridge that connects where you are and where you want to be. Most people don't think twice about developing a strategic plan for their businesses, but I will venture a guess that most people do not think about developing a strategic plan for their lives—especially their late lives. People who embrace AgePotential realize that having a life plan goes hand in hand with the power to live a fulfilling, self-directed life, and therefore they readily map out a compelling future.

Developing a plan is not a one-time event, however. Annual reviews are required, and decade milestone birthdays are another natural time for reevaluation. Like Jeff, are you implementing a strategic plan that gives you direction for today and increases your potential for tomorrow?

Laurie Robinson
Age 60

You don't describe the world you see. You see the world you describe. —Michael Beckwith

Just as the quote above suggests, if you give two people with similar circumstances the opportunity to describe their world from their own perspectives, the results can be dramatically different. The following scenarios have derived from two fifty-something women, both recently widowed, independent, financially secure, and with three children who are all out of the home. Each has a distinctly different slant on life when asked, "Describe your current reality."

Scenario one: "I cannot believe all the crap one has to put up with these days! I can't turn on the television without sponsors in my face, selling pure junk for top dollar. Work has been out of control, and I don't have time to take care of myself anymore. When I get home at the end of a long day, I don't want to move! In fact, I am so sick and tired of dealing with cranky people all day, I'd rather stay home where I can call the shots. It's a relief to have my kids grown because all they want from me is money. I've had it! I just want to be left alone!"

Scenario two: "Life has been so good to me. Every morning when I awaken, it's a gift. It's getting increasingly difficult to get in my exercise regimen with the demands of my work schedule. But I have come to realize that if I don't take care of myself now, I am prone to being unhealthy in my senior years. I value the legacy I leave for my children, so I have decided to be more intentional in my relationships with them and others. Though I dislike all the pressures around me, I have decided to let go of the things beyond my control and tackle only things within my control. Though my kids are grown and out of the house, I am so blessed to have their support as I transition into the next phase of my life. It never ceases to amaze me how life can feel so overwhelming at times, but then good people breathe reality into my circumstances, and I find resilience through the hardships. I'm blessed beyond measure."

How can two individuals, whose profiles and career paths parallel each other, be so dramatically different? One exhibits bitterness, negativity, and rebellion, and the other models hopefulness, gratitude, and optimism. Attitude can make or break the future. Those who live intentionally and are mindful that there are a multitude of choices tied to each circumstance seem to live with greater contentment. In fact, Chuck Swindoll affirms that attitude is only 10 percent of what actually happens in life and 90 percent of how one responds to it.

I am so grateful to view my own life scenario from the more positive perspective. Dr. Michael Fullan, an international change agent in the world of education, states that "Actions precede belief and buy-in." If these words indeed are true, then active life lessons are worth sharing from my years spent as a wife, mother, educator, and most recently a widow.

As a curious person, I have always had a deep passion for experiencing as many things as I can. I love movement...music...taking risks...meeting new people...traveling to interesting places. What I have concluded is that I can learn from any and all experiences, but personal change occurs when I quiet myself and take intentional time to *reflect up*on what I've learned from the experience. In the reflection, I get the "value-added" experience.

Nothing rings more true than experiencing the recent losses of multiple family members (eleven total) in a very short period of time. And they occurred in the most peculiar order, nearly all of them from youngest to oldest, and at rapid fire! What I know now is that there is *gain* in loss. But it has its very ugly stages of wrestling and working itself out. And for a person who likes to be proactive, the timetable to wholeness never happens quickly enough.

Most of my life, I have had the liberty of choice. But death doesn't seem part of that bargain. It is far beyond my boundaries to control. In retrospect, these loved ones were not put on the planet to complete my life! But because I feel so deeply about my relationships and my experiences, these departures were extremely taxing on my emotional well-being.

All of us share a common story as we expect loved ones in our lives to die. But for our family, the good-byes began first with five unexpected young adults—a niece, a nephew, two brothers, and a sister-in-law. Then followed the expected deaths of my father and mother, my grandmother, and father-in-law. Next, the devastating departure of our niece's five-year-old daughter, who discovered a loaded gun on a desk at a friend's home, which ended her life. The cycle of death for our family didn't seem to stop. But *nothing* prepared me for the swift departure of my very best friend—my husband.

We had just returned from the Galapagos, where we celebrated our thirty-sixth anniversary and had a fantastic time of love and recommitment. Neil had left the heavy demands of his investment business, and I had taken a needed reprieve from my district position as a curriculum specialist. After returning home, Neil said, "Laurie, with the departure of six family members in the last fifteen months, we really should talk about our own departures. Today, I'd die a happy man! In fact, honey, if I could choose a way to die, it would be quickly and with a basketball in my hands."

Three weeks later, I returned home from training a Denver school district, and we grabbed a bite to eat. As Neil left for basketball, he cupped my cheek in such an endearing way and said, "I love you." Later that evening, I received a call that he had collapsed from a heart attack and, just as he requested, *he died quickly and with a basketball in his hands.*

Neil—a handsome, fit, active man of fifty-six— suffered a massive heart attack without any noticeable precursor symptoms. This horrific event completely blew the wind out of my sails! Though I was a successful educator, what was my personal life going to be like without the other half of my heart? I didn't know where God was taking me, yet I knew His path would be revealed in time.

Shortly after the funeral, a dear friend stopped by the house to take a walk and pray with me. I said, "I just can't believe how quickly these past five days have gone by." My friend replied, "Laurie, this is day eleven, honey. Let's get you showered and out for some fresh air and a good walk!"

This personal journey has been the most difficult path I have yet experienced. In my deepest reflective circumstances, although I remember nearly all the painful yet healthy stages of grief, the one emotion that did not overtake me was anger. I have had a plethora of sad and dark times, but never have I had my fists pumping my pillow or, worse yet, blaming God for "doing" this to me.

Actually, the only moments I can recall with some anger were hearing the voices of well-meaning people telling me my life will never be the same: "Being a widow is a tough lot, Laurie. Not very many people fill that void at your age in life." What angered me the most was the limited, debilitated thinking behind that statement. It's a lie! In fact, I would be as bold to say that kind of thinking is simply bull! It will only come to fruition if I limit myself to thinking life can't go on with purpose any longer.

But it can! There *is*, most assuredly, gain in pain. It's the pits to go through it, but it has a refining, cleansing, polishing effect. As I now see it, I have been "broken open" to be more than I ever was: to feel more deeply, more genuinely, and with greater empathy for those around me.

It has been three years since Neil's departure, and I love him more today than ever before. It's all about reflection. I have now gotten to a place where I have *chosen* to see the blessed gift of the years we spent as a team, and I want to share those memories with my grandchildren and other loved ones as I continue to steep in the reflection and mature from the loss. The chord of three strands is hard to unravel. Yet confidently God has my future in his hands and I live expectantly, intentionally, and with great gratitude for each breath.

I have been an educator all my life. One year prior to Neil's death, I had been invited to be a national trainer for a company out of Bloomington, Indiana. In reflection, I now see that God was preparing me for keeping my head and heart busy as a passionate instructor in Neil's absence. In the past three years, I have been in thirty-four states and three foreign countries, training schools in "best practices" in education. God knew what I needed to establish a "new normal" as a single. I have had to claw my way to health and wellness—the hardest work I have ever done, but the deepest and most meaningful to date. And God continues to open doors as I open myself to His leading.

The Almighty is "repurposing" me, and I find myself stronger and more mature and resilient than ever before! Rather than mourning over "what was," I now have a new vision of "what will be." However, I am able to rejoice today and revisit the beauty of my married life with Neil, absent of regret or sadness. We have raised three beautiful children, who are happy, healthy, and successful as they train up their families for a life of love and service. This rejuvenates me, and I also find great contentment knowing my professional work is impacting twenty-first-century education. I am choosing wholeness!

To take devastation and develop a new passion that gives joy, fulfillment, direction, and renewed purpose—I have *learned and grown* from the death experience. In fact, I am hopeful that my life experience can be used to help others who have walked a similar path and need to know wholeness is emerging in those who dare to reach for it. God's words reiterate hopefulness for all who have been broken: "Being confident of this, He who began a good work in you, will carry it on to completion" (Philippians 1:6).

....

Resilience . . .
Sometimes we learn the best lessons in life when we find our own solutions, rather than when we simply do what society models for us.

Laurie willingly and courageously chose to grow while enduring the pain, darkness, and devastation of losing the love of her life. This resilience helped her move through the pain to arrive at a renewed sense of life and purpose. Laurie's deepest moment of pain never overtook her hope and belief in the possibility of a bright future.

Thrivers are able to move on, to let go of the past, and to anticipate an even better future. More importantly, they tend to savor past experiences and feel grateful for them, instead of lamenting for what's gone. Laurie embodies this sentiment: "Tis better to have loved and lost than never to have loved at all."

When challenged or distressed, resilient people expect to find a way to make things work. They feel capable and self-reliant and have a learning/coping response instead of a victim/blaming reaction. The key to resilience is the ability to cope, to ask for help, to maintain a positive attitude, and to take action even in the face of adversity. The stronger and more resilient you are, the better your chances of weathering the challenges that come your way.

There is much to lose in this world, but there is one thing that cannot be stripped from us: the inherent self-worth within us all. Laurie, after a period of deep contemplation, came to understand that "these loved ones were not put on the planet to complete my life!" We can still find purpose and meaning in our lives, regardless of our losses or change in life circumstances.

Fear results if we resist the uncertainty before us. Laurie fearlessly embraced the unknown of her future and was open to see new aspects of herself. Laurie refused to take on society's limited vision of what life must be like after losing a loved one: "The Almighty is 'repurposing' me, and I find myself stronger and more mature and resilient than ever before! Rather than mourning over 'what was,' I now have a new vision of 'what will be.'" Living a life dedicated to intentional reflection serves Laurie well; it is her source of strength. What's more, the solitude she finds through her faith appears to be the foundation of her resilience.

As we age, we are constantly reminded that this body, this life, is temporary. When we come face to face with our mortality, as Laurie did through the death of many of her loved ones, we are thrown upon our spiritual resources. In fact, our "spiritual health" may be measured by how we perceive our own mortality. In her book *The Gift of Years,* Joan Chittister points out that "Age is the antidote to personal destruction, the call to spiritual growth, because age finally brings us to the point where there is nowhere else to go but inside for comfort, inside for wealth, inside for the things that really count." Laurie's deep faith is a strong inner resource that has shaped her resilient worldview.

Loss and hardship are an inescapable part of life and often arrive without warning. How will you, like Laurie, nurture your inner resources of resilience today to help you overcome the challenges of tomorrow?

Salvador Valdovinos
Age 87

From an early age, I quickly learned how to overcome adversity to become a survivor. As a young Mexican immigrant, I endured many obstacles that became the catalyst for me to develop a life-enhancing strategy of focusing on my goals and not my circumstances.

Born October 25, 1925, I emigrated from Mexico to Milwaukee, Wisconsin, at the age of five. I wanted to be very "American" and remember looking in the mirror at age fourteen, envisioning myself with blond hair and blues eyes, only to realize I was brown eyed, dark skinned, and dark haired—just how a Mexican boy should look. I came to be okay with that.

As a kid, I was always taking care of my brothers, and I also took good care of myself. My parents instilled in me a deep sense of responsibility for the safety of my brothers and myself. I really never put myself in harm's way. My intuition told me to stay away from harmful activities, but yet I still felt open to explore and had a curiosity for life.

Being the only Mexican family in the neighborhood, others kids often teased me with insulting, hurtful words, saying I was dumb. But my saving grace was the story I told myself: "They really don't know me. If they knew me, they wouldn't say those things." My intuition told me not to believe their words. Instead, I chose to befriend them, and friends we became.

In school, I loved learning English, and I saved my money to take classical trumpet lessons. At the end of fifth grade, I received my report card informing me that I was being "retained." My teacher told me I hadn't failed but needed a better understanding of the material. I continued on with my education, only to be "retained" again in seventh grade. This time, my teacher told me, "You are doing the best you can, and that's all you can do." To this day, I always do my best.

Not long after that, I was sent to trade school to learn welding and carpentry, never finishing high school. My teacher, Ms. Stevenson, was concerned I wouldn't be able to make a living for myself and that I would end up on welfare, so she assured me trade school was a good thing. I liked Ms. Stevenson, and I trusted her recommendation because she really knew me, unlike the boys who teased me and called me "dumb." She was concerned about my life and was well intended. It ended up being the best of all worlds for me: I am now a tradesman and I am educated.

At age eighteen, I entered the army, replacing my trumpet with a rifle. In the midst of combat in WWII, my commander gave me a cigarette, telling me it would "calm my nerves," but all I did was cough invariably for ten minutes. That was my first and last cigarette, which affirmed my belief that I know what's best for me. I now take short naps and meditate each morning and evening to quiet my mind, which otherwise is like a chatterbox. I find myself better able to focus and be more productive.

Returning from the war, I was told I was a bright young man and encouraged to go to college on the GI Bill. I completed my first year at the University of Wisconsin, only to find out I had failed every class and was asked to leave. Determined to obtain my degree, I asked the counselor if I could return once I gained the necessary skills for college. I went to night school to study basic grammar and writing skills, while I worked as a welder during the day. By this time, I was married and had one child.

Upon returning to college, the counselor stated, "You're back—nobody really comes back." My response was, "I want this degree, and I'll stay until I finish." I graduated with a BA in sociology with a scholarship for graduate school. I went on to obtain an MA in psychology from the University of Indiana. I returned to Milwaukee to thank Ms. Stevenson for all her encouragement and to share my accomplishments, but she had died.

Degree in hand, I launched my own practice, Life Management Institute, teaching people how to create, manage, and live their best lives. Life is a balancing act, and to maintain a healthy flow, all areas need to be in harmony: relationships, health and well-being, time management, personal development, values and goals, and finances.

Through years of observation, I realized the more attention a person gives to a behavior they want to release, the stronger the behavior's hold seems to be. What proves to be the most promising way to affect change is simply being aware of the need to change and using it as a springboard for a new vision and plan of action. I often prescribed my clients to give TEA Time: Time, Energy, and Attention to the new life they now desired to create and live. In my personal and professional experience, the individuals who struggle the most with creating positive, healthy change are those who lack the willingness and openness to do what it takes to say yes to the opportunities that will promote or further the life they want to create. These individuals readily say yes to the intention but not the action.

I would not be able to teach these concepts and techniques if I, myself, didn't believe and practice them. I retired in 1990 with a sense of knowing that I, in a small way, empowered people to live their *best* lives.

Since then, I have been certified as a coach, and I work out of my home, incorporating many of the concepts and techniques I found to be successful in my practice. At eighty-six, I continue to coach clients onsite as well as on Skype and over the telephone. I receive a lot of joy from my work. It is very gratifying to have clients tell me they have learned and grown so much that they choose to pass on the empowering information to their children and grandchildren.

In 2009, I lost the love of my life to an eight-year battle of multiple myeloma cancer. Olga, my second wife, was like a soul mate to me. I became her caretaker over those years, often engaging in conversations about death and dying and the life she wanted me to have after her passing. This proved to be very therapeutic and has helped me move through the grieving process and let her go.

The wisdom my father shared with me on the day I left to serve in the war has become my foundation for how I overcome pain, loss, death, and hardship of any kind. He told me, "As a soldier, you are going to have to kill the enemy, so do so in service for your country—or the enemy will kill you. After you are done, leave the memories there." As I put the meaning of his words together, I realized that at any moment I could be killed; therefore, I shouldn't waste energy thinking about dying, but instead put that energy into living. I took his advice. I came home and put my energy and attention toward creating and living a new life, never experiencing any posttraumatic stress, as many do. Acknowledge the painful experience, reflect on it to learn the lessons and gain the benefits, and then let go and move on. Our spouses, children, grandchildren, and professions all enhance our lives, but they cannot be our purpose to live and live abundantly, because they can all be gone in a flash.

I have always felt responsible for my own health and well-being. I believe my genes have less influence on how I age than my thoughts, attitudes, and lifestyle do. Exercise, diet, meditation, and my spiritual practice of gratitude are priorities in managing my health. I was diagnosed with prostate cancer in 1989, but I never let the disease define me or limit me. I intentionally put my thoughts on healing and regaining full health. I went through radioactive seed treatment, and I have been cancer free ever since. And because diabetes runs in my family, I keep myself at a healthy weight.

I am eighty-seven years young and don't *feel* "old"

at all. Although at age fifty, I thought people in their eighties were old. I really didn't understand what it meant to live on the other side of fifty. I can tell you there is a lot of hope, joy, and fulfillment ahead, but you must choose life over the loss and disappointments. Chances are, people who dread growing older are probably not very satisfied or fulfilled in the present moment. I have learned to live a fulfilling life out of choice, not out of my circumstances.

I am here to be of service to my fellow human beings. I have always wanted to live my life being robust and fully active up until the day I die. At the moment, my greatest joys are my grandchildren, carpentry work, pen making, socializing, coaching clients, speaking engagements, teaching opportunities, and being in Toastmasters. I have many meaningful things I still want to tackle: writing a book, becoming a professional speaker (actually getting paid), and who knows, maybe finding another "love of my life"!

....

Self-Efficacy, Mastery…

Do you ever hear people use the past as an excuse for the present, saying, "I had a tough childhood, and so that's why…" Well, not Sal. He never allowed adversity to deter him from pursuing his dreams. At a young age, Sal developed a coping mechanism that continues to serve him today. He learned that if he focused on his goals and what he ultimately wanted out of life, he could forge on and avoid being defeated by his circumstances.

This coping mechanism is based on a concept called self-efficacy, which is a person's belief in his or her ability to succeed in a particular situation. According to psychologist Albert Bandura, self-efficacy plays a major role not only in how people think, behave, and feel, but also in how people determine goals, tasks, and challenges.

Sal chose to learn from the criticism he received and failure he experienced early on, and he created an emotional strategy to protect his inner self-worth. As a result, he empowered himself to overcome many significant challenges. He did not expect someone to rescue him or make excuses for him; instead, he exerted his own power by reframing his hurtful childhood experiences. For example, Sal told himself, "They really don't know me. If they knew me, they wouldn't say those things." Verbal encouragement from his parents and especially from a special teacher helped Sal overcome self-doubt at a critical time.

During his childhood, Sal developed a deep inner confidence and learned to rely on his inner wisdom over the advice of others. For example, by age eighteen, Sal had developed enough confidence in himself to disregard his commander's advice to smoke in order to alleviate anxiety. He decided that smoking was not in his best interest, and he continues to make good choices for himself today.

People who have a higher self-efficacy perceive fewer barriers or are less influenced by them. Efficacious people tend to approach more challenging tasks, work harder, and have a persistent nature even in the face of early failures. Setbacks didn't seem to deter Sal. He remained persistent and confident that he would eventually succeed. Those lacking self-efficacy often won't even attempt to start a new challenge, or they will quit at the earliest sign of difficulty.

As Sal exemplifies, the concept of self-efficacy can be applied to all areas of life. It is what gets a person through the day and through tough times. Sal and all other thrivers have an individual belief that their choices and actions will determine the outcomes in their lives. Gerontologists call this concept mastery. Over time, Sal's small successes built upon one another, gradually strengthening his self-confidence and helping him cope and overcome adversity, and that resulted in a life strategy of personal mastery.

According to Sal, a fulfilling life is not based on life circumstances, but on choice. What new choices will you make today that will lead you to mastery, just like Sal?

A New Vision of Aging

I hope you now have a greater awareness of the fact you can establish a new perspective on aging—one free from stereotypes, socialization, and fear. However, you must believe the possibility to be true for yourself and then act on that new belief. Real transformation cannot take place overnight; instead, it requires long-term, daily cultivation. There is purpose in aging. Many people view growing old as a gift full of unforeseen pleasures, and you can, too. In fact, I don't know any-one who *doesn't* want to live a healthy, adventure-filled, meaningful life until his or her dying day.

You now know your later years are full of potential to evolve, grow, contribute, and live a purposeful, pas-sionate life. And so I ask: *Are you willing to believe it is possible for you? And are you willing to commit to creating and living it? If not now, then when?*

Let us now *refocus* our time, energy, and attention from the dreaded *D*s—dependence, disease, disability, despair, depression, denial, and decline—to a new vision of aging. You can start by doing the following actions:

Relinquishing what doesn't serve you.

Rewiring your brain for mindful, present-moment living.

Rethinking what it means to age.

Reflecting on becoming whole, not old.

Retreating inwardly in order to outwardly express your deepest passions and truest self.

Rekindling your youthful enthusiasm and passion for life.

Repurposing the energy you spend worrying, putting it instead toward pursuing your passions.

Reenvisioning yourself to reflect who you are today, not yesterday.

Realigning your thoughts with my new concept of aging. Think *aging*, think *potential*. Think AgePotential!

Now you can tap into the potentiality of life. Remember, it's your life and your potential. No matter your age, you can begin to see each moment as an opportunity to create a better world. The big challenge, according to Richard Rohr, author of *Falling Upward*, "is to become all that you have the possibility of becoming. You cannot believe what it does to the human spirit to maximize your human potential and stretch yourself to the limit." Indeed, our bodies are all growing older in chronological years, but our spirits are ageless and alive, looking for the next adventure.

Living beyond the status quo—beyond the socialization and stereotypes—and reclaiming your full vitality is both your individual right and our collective responsibility. By embracing the possibility of AgePotential and believing you can become a *thriver*, you will join an empowered minority. The time for passivity is gone. Now is the time to *awaken* to the opportunity to either become part of the solution or part of the problem.

So raise your awareness. Raise your standards. Fight for a robust and healthy mind, body, and spirit. And never back down.

Now, go and live out your AgePotential!

Contributor Biographies

Milt "Beaver" Adams

The life of Milt "Beaver" Adams took many interesting turns. After a fifteen-year career in corporate America, he launched himself to be the maverick entrepreneur he was always destined to become. After many years as a solopreneur in the marketing, advertising, and printing business, Milt founded Beaver's Pond Press in 1998 at age seventy. When asked why he would undertake such a big project at that time of his life, he chuckled and said, "It's my destiny and my passion. All my life's experiences, both business and personal, have led me to this adventure." Milt lives in Edina, Minnesota with his wife, Jean, and his King Charles cavalier spaniel, Chloe. More information can be found about Milt at www.beaverspondpress.com.

Lynette Crane

Lynette Crane, MA, is a certified life coach and a Minneapolis-based speaker, writer, and coach who specializes in helping overly busy women expand their time and find "islands of peace" in their daily lives from which to create a "juicy" life, even when they think they don't have the time to do so. Lynette is the author of *Stop Your Stress Now!*, *The Confident Introvert: Gain the Skills to Overcome Shyness and Low Self-Esteem*, an audio self-coaching program called *30 Steps to Serenity*, and an audio relaxation program called *A Journey to Your Islands of Peace*. Lynette Crane can be found at www.CreativeLifeChanges.com.

Nadia Giordana

Author and lifestyle strategist Nadia Giordana focuses her energies on helping women in midlife find the courage or inspiration they need to rediscover their sidelined dreams and go out and do the things they always said they were going to do. She can be reached at her website, www.embodyyourvision.com. Nadia is author of the books *Thinking Skinny* and *Reinventing New Chapters in Your Life at Any Age*.

Connie Goldman

Formerly on the staff of National Public Radio, Connie Goldman was an award-winning radio producer and reporter. For over thirty years she has been exclusively concerned with the changes and challenges of aging in America. Her presentations are designed to inform, empower, and inspire. Connie's books include *Who Am I Now That I'm Not Who I Was?* and *The Gifts of Caregiving: Stories of Hardship, Hope, and Healing.* www.congoldman.org

Fran Heitzman

In 1987, Fran Heitzman founded Bridging while he was the maintenance man at Pax Christi Church in Eden Prairie, Minnesota. After finding a nonprofit that was thrilled to receive a crib that wasn't needed in the church nursery, Fran thought he could do the same thing for other essential items, too. Thus, Bridging was born. Since then, Bridging has become the largest furniture bank in North America and will serve its sixty thousandth family in July 2012. Fran continues to volunteer at Bridging and has received many honors for his service, including the MetLife Foundation's Older Volunteers Enrich America Award. More information can be found at www.bridging.org.

Jerry Johncock

Jerry Johncock was born February 2, 1928 to Esther and Lynden Johncock. After completing two years college (1947–1948), he served in the US Navy (1948–1952). In 1949 in Boston, God called him to evangelize. In 1953 he married Dorlene Ramey, and together they held revivals in Michigan, Mexico, and Trinidad. Before marriage, he told Dorlene that he wanted five boys for a basketball team. Thomas was born in 1955, then James, Philip, William, and last Mark in 1966, and they praised Jesus for such a wonderful family. Jerry started running at age fifty after his three younger sons talked him into it and has been running ever since. So far, he has run 114 marathons, but hopes to compete in 200 by the end of his running career. Jerry can be reached at tjjohncock@yahoo.com.

Marjorie Johnson

Marjorie Johnson, author of the cookbook *The Road to Blue Ribbon Baking with Marjorie*, is the winner of over one thousand blue ribbons for her baking at the Minnesota State and Anoka County fairs. A frequent guest on local and national television including *The Tonight Show with Jay Leno*, *The Dr. Oz Show*, *The Martha Stewart Show*, *The Rosie O'Donnell Show*, and *The*

View, Marjorie entertains viewers with her enthusiasm, energy, and passion for baking. Married to husband Lee for over sixty-five years, they have three grown children. With a degree in home economics from the University of Minnesota, Marjorie is a true proponent of healthy eating and daily exercise. Marjorie can be reached at www.blueribbonbaking.com.

Jeff Noel
Boomer, husband, dad, speaker, runner, servant. Orlando resident Jeff Noel gratefully and humbly travels the world as a professional speaker for Disney Institute. In 2009 at age fifty, what began as a one hundred-day challenge to leave a trail for his young son in case something bad ever happened to himself has morphed into a personal mission to challenge 3 percent of baby boomers to do something great before they die. With seven thousand + blog posts on Life's Five Big Choices, Jeff has become America's unheralded work-life balance expert. You can easily find Jeff Noel by Googling his name or by visiting MidLifeCelebration.com.

Laurie Robinson

Laurie Robinson is president of ((((EduPulse Consulting)))), an international consulting company specializing in educational best practices. Additionally, Laurie trains teachers and administrators across America and abroad through two premier professional development companies: Solution Tree and Marzano Research Laboratory. In addition, Ms. Robinson facilitates strategic planning with an emphasis on vision planning and collaborative culture development. As a passionate practitioner, Laurie works directly with classroom teachers to develop engaging tasks to prepare the twenty-first century learner. Laurie is "button-popping-proud" of her three children, Aaron, Heather, and Carson, and three grandchildren, Avi, Alia, and Halle. She resides in suburban Minneapolis, Minnesota. To connect with Laurie, please email her at Laurie.7robinson@gmail.com.

Salvador J. Valdovinos

Salvador J. Valdovinos, MA, is a psychologist, coach, speaker, consultant, and founder of Life Management Institute, Inc. An accomplished psychologist of a professional practice of fifty-two years, Sal is capitalizing on his life experience and is committed to helping people to create, live, and manage their own best life. At eighty-seven years of age, Sal is grateful for his excellent health and well-being. In Sal's mind, his capabilities are just as potent as when he was young. He continues to work out of his home coaching clients through Skype and teleconference. Sal can be reached at sjvaldovinos@comcast.net.

AgePotential™ Resources

Join our AgePotential community and connect with like-minded people who aspire to thrive to their highest potential for their whole lives long.

Facebook Fan Page:
www.facebook.com/GenerationAgePotential

Twitter: @AgePotential

YouTube: www.youtube.com/AgePotential

LinkedIn:
www.linkedin.com/in/loriacampbell

Pinterest: www.pinterest.com/AgePotential

We also suggest you visit www.agepotential.com and take the FREE AgePotential Quiz and sign up to receive FREE weekly aging affirmations.

Start Living Your AgePotential Today!
We're here to *support* you in creating a life in which you **thrive** at every age and stage in life. Accelerate your path to living your BEST life by making a commitment to act on your intention and get involved:

Facilitate Deeper Discussion and Reflection
Go to www.agepotential.com and sign up to receive a FREE Digging Deeper Kit in which you will be able to download a series of thought-provoking questions conducive for book club or individual use. Included is an added BONUS of a MP3 of the profiled thrivers posing their own questions to you!

Join an AgePotential Mastermind Group
If you are interested in creating positive, healthy change in your life or desire to engage with like-

minded aspiring thrivers, this is the group for you! For more details and benefits of such a group, email info@agepotential.com or visit www.agepotential .com/mastermind-group/.

Bring Lori Campbell to Your Organization

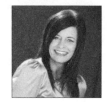

Lori, the voice of AgePotential, will educate, inspire, and empower your audience to *thrive* and much, much more! For more details, email info@ agepotential.com or visit www.age potetial.com/speaking.